Okay, I quit.
Now what?

Becoming a
Re-Invented Alcoholic

By:

Mark A. Tuschel

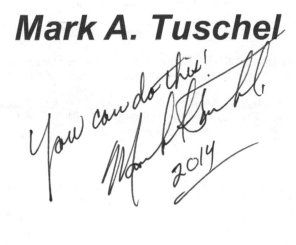

Legal Mumbo Jumbo

Okay I quit. Now what?

Becoming a Re-Invented Alcoholic.

Published by: CW Media, Inc.

Proudly printed in the United States of America

All inquiries about this book, including interviews, purchases or speaking engagements can be made through email: **booksales@LivingSoberSucks.com**

Please do not bother contacting the Library of Congress Cataloging-in-Publication Data. They have enough problems of their own and they're pretty busy from what I hear.

ISBN 13: 978-0-9842730-3-4

Dedication:

"To you.
I don't know you and you don't know me,
but you have helped me. Thank you."

Mark A. Tuschel

"I understand that I will not get all that I want, but I will make my best effort to make it all happen. I will also be prepared to adapt my schedule and my life to conditions, but I will NOT adapt or compromise my core principles. There are things that I want in life and this is why I will stay sober. It is up to ME to stick to my plan and make the things I plan happen in my life."

Mark A. Tuschel

Table of contents

Introduction:

S topping destructive drinking can be the easy part, but what do you do tonight, tomorrow, this weekend, when you go on vacation, for the rest of your life? That is the hard part. This book will hopefully help you discover some of those answers.

If all you want to do is stay sober, then simply lock yourself in your own home or apartment. Create your own self-imposed prison. Don't go anywhere. Don't go out. Don't go to parties, events, sports, music, entertainment or social gatherings. You can also insulate yourself from the rest of the world by surrounding yourself with only "program" people or people from your exclusive sober club. You can do that if you wish, but you're only robbing yourself (and possibly others who are close to you) of a fully exciting and interesting world that is available to each of us.

The act of drinking requires time. Not just pouring a drink into your mouth, but all the hours which revolve around it. Sitting around with other drunks at a bar, sitting at home staring at the TV, drinking and shooting the breeze with neighbors or friends, whatever. Most of us drink and don't do much of anything else while we're drinking. Oh sure, we might be doing chores or working on a project, but drinking really does require focused attention and TIME. Then of course there's the time afterwards or the next day to recover from our previous day or night of drinking.

Once that act is eliminated from your life, you're left with a lot of time on your hands. So now what do you do with that time? This is going to be a process of discovery. Discovering what you find interesting and what things bring you joy.

If you were once a drunk, sobriety can be a difficult existence, because you will have to approach problems, human interactions, socializing and entertainment through a clear mind. Sobriety brings with it a clarity of reality and personal limitations.

Maybe you've only been sober for one day, maybe five years. This book is for the person who has already quit drinking. I'm not going to try and persuade you to quit, I don't give a shit what you do – YOU have to give a shit about what you do.

Polished psychobabble and an expansive vocabulary are pretty, but there's nothing pretty about being a slave to alcohol. So I'm going to speak in simple, straightforward terms. This book can get raw, crude or profane – as are most drunks. You might disagree with many of my philosophies. And you know what? That's great! Because that means that *YOU* are thinking on your own behalf.

This book is not the final answer to all questions about sober living. It is written based upon my own personal experiences and the input and experiences of thousands of other Re-Invented Alcoholics. I have had the joy of being able to interview and befriend many of these people. Writing this book and working with other former drunks is beneficial to me. I get to learn techniques to enjoy my own sobriety more and I get to learn from thousands of other Re-Invented Alcoholics.

Notice that there are 12 Chapters of, *Okay, I quit. Now what?* That isn't irony, I planned it that way. I like to call these, "The 12 Alternative Steps for the Re-Invented Alcoholic."

We can spend our entire lives searching and waiting. Waiting for the day that everything comes together and everything is perfect, then we'll be happy. Why wait? As a good friend of mine said, "It's never too early to start." Don't wait. – **Mark Tuschel**

#1) Facing reality

"It's never too early to start." – Jeff K.

W hat reality do you have to face? The reality that YOU no longer drink. You might tell yourself, "I'll never drink again." But some people don't like to think in "never" terms, so instead maybe you tell yourself, "I'm not going to drink today, tomorrow or in the near future." You could also say, "I'm not going to drink indefinitely." However you want to say it to yourself, the reality is that YOU no longer drink. You don't need to add qualifiers like, "I can't" or "I shouldn't" drink. Simply accept the fact that YOU no longer drink.

Don't worry about anyone else, just worry about YOU. That's another part of sober reality – other people can and will continue to drink, some socially, some to excess, some to death. That's not your problem, it's theirs. The sooner you accept this reality the sooner you will stop feeling as if you have been singled out to suffer. You won't be as tempted to look down at anyone else who does drink and you won't feel compelled to spread the "good word" of sobriety to everyone you meet.

Here are more realities that you will inevitably face: temptation, self-doubt and self-pity. Anger, guilt, frustration and sadness. Feelings of loneliness and isolation; like you're the odd person in a group or party. The dissolution of friendships and relationships. Excess time on your hands and unspent money in your pocket. Feelings of superiority, boredom, a lack of enthusiasm. These are just a few realities you're likely to encounter. I'm sure there will be others that I haven't mentioned that you will experience.

11

Some would say that many of these items that I term as *realities* are emotions or conditions which are clinical symptoms of depression. If you're being treated for depression you probably exhibit many of those traits, but every former drunk is not clinically depressed. As a Re-Invented Alcoholic you will, at some point in your life, struggle with temptation, be angry, have unspent money in your pocket and be bored – but that doesn't mean you're suffering from depression. I believe that we former drunks feel these emotions differently than someone who suffers from depression. I consider them *realities* that must be faced up to and dealt with for the rest of our sober lives. So allow me to briefly touch on the *realities* I just listed.

Temptation: There is no question that you will inevitably encounter moments of temptation, unless of course you've locked yourself away into your own prison or refuse to engage with the rest of the world. At some point you're going to be somewhere and you're going to feel like drinking. An event will occur in your life (good or bad) and you'll feel like drinking. Many functions pre-pour or set out glasses and bottles of wine. Just because complimentary champagne is offered at a wedding reception doesn't mean you have to grab a glass. You can toast with your water goblet or coffee cup. You never know when someone is innocently going to offer you a drink, or worse, someone who's drunk will push a drink on you. "Aw c'mon you pussy, you can have one drink. It's my birthday, c'mon. What's the matter with you?" Those are the dicey moments, the few seconds where you can still say, "no thanks."

Accept the reality that temptation will come at the most peculiar and inconvenient times. A lot of former drunks talk about "triggers." An aroma, a song, an activity, event or certain people can *trigger* your temptation to drink. You may not know why these *triggers* hit. Some are obvious triggers, for example you're at a wine tasting party or a beer guzzling contest. Other times triggers will come out of nowhere at the least expected moment. You need to always have your own reminder statements ready in your head. Not that you walk around constantly repeating a mantra, just have them ready because temptation is inevitable. Here are a few examples of reminder statements for you to keep in your mind. Naturally you want to come up with some on your own or special ones that resonate with you.

"Drinking right now will NOT make my life better in the future."

"I promised myself, I can't let myself down."

"Don't do it, you know better."

"This too shall pass."

"I will NOT let the motherfuckers win."

(The last one happens to be my favorite.)

Self preservation mantras are only one part of controlling temptations. The reality is that you might have to remove yourself from an event and leave the tempting environment. That's right, you might have to leave a party early or walk away from a group of people. Plan ahead and bring your own car so you can leave when you want. If you don't have your own car or can't get a ride with a sober friend then you might have to pass on some invitations – that's the reality.

Self-doubt and self-pity: These thoughts will also be inevitable, especially when you're feeling lonely or you have to pass on some tempting invitations. Every time shit doesn't turn out as you had hoped, you will be plagued by these feelings. "My friends all abandoned me, my kids still disobey me, my wife/husband/partner has become distant from me. Was this really worth it?"

When almost anything goes wrong in life, you'll think of some reason, some twisted logic to correlate your getting sober as the cause of this situation. Then you'll doubt your decision and feel sorry for yourself. But if you stop and look for the real causes, you will likely see that your sobriety has nothing to do with it or that the situation would have been far worse if this particular event took place and you were still drinking.

There will be some situations that are directly related or linked to your sobriety. The ending of friendships or relationships is one example (I'll touch on this shortly). Factual periods of loneliness and missing old friends are real, and can get you doubting your decision to live sober. But please remember that if these friendships ended because you no longer drink, were these true friendships? Why would you want to live a life of self-destruction just to keep someone as a friend?

Self-pity typically arises when you see other people drinking. "How come they can drink and I can't?" Well, you could drink, you have every legal right to do so, but will it make your life better? Will drinking get you closer to your goals and what you want out of life? Will drinking bring you closer to the friends and relationships that you really care about?

Feelings of self-doubt and self-pity are natural. Accept that these feelings will occur and at times they will cross your mind. Have positive affirmations ready to think about. Remind yourself of the reasons why you sobered up in the first place. Force yourself to recall all of the good things that have come about and all of the bad things that you have undoubtedly avoided due to your sobriety. It may be helpful for you to make a list of all the bad things you have avoided and that have left your life since you quit drinking and refer to it when you're feeling self-doubt.

Regardless of whether you're drunk or sober, every plan and desire will not come to fruition – that's just a reality. Consider all the other people in this world who don't get everything or anything they hope for. While that doesn't change your personal situation, it can help you overcome your feelings of self-doubt and self-pity.

Anger: You might find yourself getting angry at people who drink (including social drinkers). You find yourself getting angry at beer commercials on TV and angry at alcohol in general. This is another natural emotion, but there's nothing to validate it. This type of anger goes hand-in-hand with self-pity: "I feel sorry for myself because I can't drink, so I'll get angry at those who do."

Instead of being angry, try to see the humor in these things. Beer commercials for example. You can laugh at the humor and appreciate the creativity of the ad. You can also laugh at the reality of how *unreal* these ads are; the depictions of dopey guys getting hot women simply because they drink a certain brand of beer or that a certain beer makes them appear cooler, more coordinated and adept at sports... yeah right. Then there's all the commercials that show only cool, beautiful young people dancing while the DJ plays hip songs, or they're playing volleyball on a beach, everyone with tan, toned bodies. I know that that isn't reality. So what? I can still enjoy the good looking people in the commercial, laugh at the humor or even joke about how it isn't a reality.

When I find myself feeling anger towards others who are drinking, I stop myself and force myself to watch what is REALLY occurring. I frequently witness people progressively becoming drunker and drunker. I've seen many a happy couple turn vicious towards each other after they've both been drinking for a while. I watch the dynamics that evolve between people as they become increasingly drunker and arguments ensue. That's when I'm able to say to myself, "I'm glad I'm no longer like that. That used to be me. How sad." You might also become angry at yourself. Angry for things you have done, angry because you've been weak in the past, angry because you didn't sober up sooner. You can't change what WAS but you can change what will be.

Your anger can be used as a positive driving force. Anger is part of normal human *fight or flight* behavior. You *fight* through the urges to drink, you *fight* off destructive behaviors for your own self preservation, you *fight* for your right to be normal and go anywhere and everywhere you want. Your anger can be mustered to tell yourself, "I will not lose to alcohol, I have control over it." The *flight* part is when you leave tempting environments or avoid them altogether. You flee from unhealthy people and bad influences in your life. You take *flight* to preserve your own health.

Anger can also be used to prove to others that you are strong. I use self-directed anger to stay sober. This may sound psychologically unhealthy but it works for me. Plenty of people said, "Mark will never stay sober, he can't do it." I want to prove them wrong. I will not give anyone who does not support my sobriety or thinks that I can't stay sober the pleasure of being right. I will stay sober to prove any naysayer wrong. I don't gloat or flaunt my sober power; I simply allow them to witness it. My anger serves me, so long as I don't direct it towards any other person.

Guilt: You might feel guilty of your past behaviors. While you can't undo things that you have actually done, you can accept responsibility for them. Some things you can (metaphorically) pay restitution for, some you can never repay or repair. If it's something or someone that is important to you, then do your best to live amends. Notice that I didn't say, "make amends," but I said, "live amends." Anyone can say, "I'm sorry" and then go on acting like an asshole. How you behave now and how you behave in the future is living your amends. If you're truly sorry then you must live it.

You can offer a sincere and genuine apology. If the other person doesn't accept it, so be it. You can't be angry at them if they don't accept your apology. Your apology doesn't erase what you may have done (or what they think you did), but you can feel good about yourself for at least making the effort. I'm not suggesting that you hide from or deny your guilt. You have to live with the knowledge of what you may have done. You can only make sure that you don't repeat the same behavior in the future. Sometimes others may try to make you feel guilty. Again, all you can do is offer an apology and attempt to make restitution. If all the other person wants to do is make you feel guilty, then you can either agree to their abuse or liberate yourself from knowing them. Feeling guilty won't make you stronger. Acceptance of reality will make you stronger.

Frustration: You will battle with multiple types of frustration. Some examples are: Why do I keep thinking about alcohol? Why isn't anything going as I planned? Why didn't I do this sooner? I want to be happier with my sobriety but I'm not. I want more, now, faster!

People often feel frustrated because they think that they're doing the "wrong" things. Don't spend so much time thinking about, "what am I doing wrong?" Spend more time thinking about, "What have I done right? What can I do that is right" and then do more of those right things. You have to analyze and consider what isn't working and what might be wrong, but you can't dwell on the wrong. Make a note of what isn't working and don't repeat it. Focus more on thinking about the right things you can do and the right things that have worked for you in the past.

When you drank, problems, frustrations and inadequacies disappeared from your mind within the time it took you to catch a buzz – but the problems, frustrations and inadequacies still existed in reality. They usually showed up again the next morning when

17

you were sober. Sobriety brings with it harsh realizations of your own personal limitations. Knowledge and acceptance of your limitations allows you to focus more on what your actual capabilities and strengths are, and then you can make the most of them. Most of us will never get everything (if anything) that we want – that's reality – but it doesn't mean that you can't try. Quite often the process of trying is just as enjoyable and memorable as the final accomplishment.

Fixing relationships, furthering your education or learning new skills all take time, but we usually want them NOW. Frustration is a natural emotion, especially when you don't get to where you want to be as fast as you want to be there. Life isn't completed in an hour – it takes as long as you are alive to complete your life. You must accept the fact that you will have to be patient with yourself and patient with others as well.

Sadness and depression: Sadness can stem from many causes such as: Missing your old friend alcohol. Missing all the excitement you thought you once had or that you actually did have. Missing certain drinking friends. Missing the sensation of getting drunk. Sobriety not turning out to be what you were told it would be or had hoped that it would be. This might surprise you and it may not make you feel any better, but people who have never had a drink or rarely drink get sad and depressed too. Sadness and depression are normal, natural human emotions. Drinking was a way to mask or avoid those emotions. Now that you're sober, you won't be able to temporarily numb them; you'll have to deal with those natural emotions in a new way.

Under normal conditions sadness comes and goes within a person's life. Sometimes you have to just accept that you are sad on a given day and it may even go on for a few days. Typically sadness will dissolve away if you stay active and busy. If it continues for an extended period of time or if it debilitates you from leading a normal life, then you have to find out what the root cause of the sadness is. You might want to seek professional counseling, therapy, a physician, a personal coach or spiritual help. Those people can help you discover your root cause of sadness, but don't expect them to bear your burden for you. You will have to be an active participant in its discovery and cure.

Trying to find a replacement for the excitement of alcohol can be destructive. Some replacements can be more detrimental to your health than drinking. Chasing after a quick substitute can lead to a substitute addiction and disappointment, which in turn will lead to more depression. Accept the reality that NOTHING can or will replace the mind and body altering sensation of getting drunk. There is nothing else like it. Accepting this may not rid you of your immediate sadness and depression, but it will help you come to terms with the reality that you no longer drink. You will then have to focus your mind on other healthy, productive and pleasant activities that *do* bring you joy. Do not seek an exact replacement for alcohol – there is NONE.

Feeling like the odd person in the group or at a party: It's natural to feel isolated when you no longer drink. When you're at a party or social gathering the only people you *see* are the ones who are drinking. If you go sit in a bar, that's what most people are doing there – drinking. However, if you go to a concert, a comedy club, sporting event, wedding reception or party, and you were to look a bit closer, you'll see that not everyone is drinking.

If you obsess about it and you're constantly watching everyone else to see who is or isn't drinking, you'll never have fun at social events and you'll never be able to interact normally. Other people who drink, that are not a part of your immediate life, **are not your problem**. Mind your own business. If it's too much of a struggle for you or you're too tempted to watch everyone else, then don't go to public events or social gatherings where alcohol is served.

Sorry, but you just gotta get over the urge to watch everyone else.

In the event you do venture out to social gatherings where alcohol is served, you can always carry a non-alcoholic drink in your hand if that helps you feel more normal. For example, I like to carry a glass of seltzer water with a twist of lemon. That way people aren't always asking me if they can get me a drink. If they do ask, I say, "No thanks', I'm fine" and I leave it at that. I don't explain anything. If they offer to buy me a shot I say, "No I'm okay." If I have to join in on a toast, I raise my glass of seltzer in celebration. If the person keeps pushing and prodding me to drink I impolitely tell them to, "fuck off and leave me alone." If you feel odd, it's only because YOU feel that way. You are not odd and if anyone tries to make you feel odd, get away from them immediately, they're not healthy for you.

The dissolution of friendships and relationships: Some friendships and relationships will end as a result of your sober lifestyle and some will end by your own choosing. If you think about it, I'm sure that you've had plenty of friendships or relationships come and go while you were a drinker. A few (if not most) probably ended in drunken arguments. But now that you're living sober, the ending of friendships seems to stand out more. We seem to miss the *memory* of how good a friendship was. If it was a friendship or relationship based predominantly on being drinking partners, then it wasn't a good friendship to begin with.

It's tempting to revisit old drinking friends because you miss them. I've done it. I've gone out with old friends and it wasn't the best experience for me. I watched as they got plowed and I felt embarrassed and sad for them. But then I felt sorry for myself. I missed *the memory* of having drunken fun with them and it quietly made me wonder, "Maybe I could go back out with them and have only a couple of drinks?" They weren't tempting me – I was tempting and teasing myself. I had to accept the reality that if a friendship isn't good for my sober health then I'm better off without it, as painful as that may be. I've found new friends and the ones that have remained have become even better friends.

Excess time on your hands: Drinking takes up a lot of time; it requires dedication and focus. Don't laugh, it does. When I drank, my every thought was planning ahead – planning how and when I could start drinking. Once I quit, I had a lot of time on my hands and I had no idea what to do with it. I'll cover this subject in greater detail in Chapters #4 & #5.

The reality of feeling bored or overwhelmed can't be avoided either. I had never seen my life through sober eyes before. Suddenly everything blatantly stood out; debt, clutter, halfhearted efforts, failed efforts, responsibilities. Having no experience at knowing what to do with all this time (and these ugly realities) made my newly undertaken sobriety even more agonizing. Sober, *time* felt like the enemy.

Initially I started attending meetings, randomly cleaning my house, doing odd projects around my house and occasionally exercising. I wanted to use up time, but I had no sense of purposeful direction so I was still bored with these activities. As I finally came to accept the reality that I was going to have a lot of time on my hands, I realized that I needed to have something purposeful to do. I didn't want to just putter along doing random busy work or go sit in meetings night after night. I wanted to harness the power of my sobriety and make my sobriety reward me. That is when I asked myself the question: "What do you want out of sobriety?" (You'll be asked this question in Chapter #2.)

When I had answers to those questions, I was able to work on my plan. Having a plan gave me focus. This completely changed the reality of excess time on my hands. Yes, I still get bored and yes, I still have excess time on my hands, but when that occurs, I can always go back to my plan for, "What do you want out of sobriety?"

Boredom: This dovetails with excess time on your hands. No doubt about it, you will get bored. I'm sure that you felt bored at times when you drank, but when you're drunk you don't notice the feeling. Even if you experience less actual *bored time* than you did when you were drinking, sober boredom will feel more intense. The reality is that it is no one else's responsibility to keep you entertained. It is no one else's responsibility to find something for you to do. You have to do things on your own. You can just sit there and be bored if you want – but sitting there, wondering what you *feel* like doing can be dangerous for your continued sobriety. Self-pity and self-doubt shows up, and sadness follows. Then what looks tempting as an easy out from boredom would be to drink again.

During the inevitable periods of boredom that will strike is when you turn to your "What do you want out of sobriety list." Checking your list will at least bring your focus back to thinking about why you want to live sober and it will remind you of things you can and should do (that's if you made a list). You can be busy as hell and still feel bored (most of us call that "having a job"). Boredom is part of human life, whether you're drunk or sober.

Unspent money in your pocket: This is a new dilemma for most drunks because you will have unspent money and you WILL have to do something with it. What are you going to do with the money you're no longer spending? If you don't have plans for it, it will migrate to an unknown invisible planet. If you never stash away what you *would have* spent on drinking, you'll miss seeing the financial benefits and never enjoy your savings. You want to be able to have some fun with it, treat yourself or do something nice for the people you care about. This will be part of the reward system that you'll develop for yourself explained in Chapter #3.

Feelings of superiority: This is a fine line that must be held. I am a firm believer in being proud of yourself, but when you cross over into a *self-righteous preacher* you are actually diminishing your own pride. You are just a normal person like everyone else; the only difference is that you are no longer a slave to alcohol.

Feelings of superiority can happen when a group of "recovered alcoholics" get together. They start talking about all the other weak and despicable drunks and begin to compliment one another on how wonderful, smart and enlightened each of them is. There's nothing wrong with sober fellowship, joking and talking about your own past foibles and gossiping about other's debacles. But a sense of humility and a gracious attitude will serve you best. This goes back to seeing old drinking friends. You may want to go "show off" your new sobriety skills. Don't do it. Bragging about your sobriety and belittling others will make you look like an arrogant asshole. And if you hang out with them long enough, you may crack and relapse – then you'll *be* an asshole.

Remember that you were just like all the drunks you see fault in, possibly even worse. Just because you saw "the light" doesn't make you a better person than someone else. It only means that you took control of your own life. Be proud of yourself and your own accomplishments regarding your sobriety. The reality is that there's always somebody who's better at something than you are.

Lack of enthusiasm: Life might feel flat and dull after you begin sobriety. Being responsible, doing what needs to be done, taking care of obligations and spending time with certain people isn't always as wildly exciting as getting drunk. But being responsible can bring you deeper, more rewarding experiences.

You can always force yourself to feign enthusiasm (women have been doing this with me for years). Seriously, forcing yourself to express interest in something or faking a bit of enthusiasm isn't shallow advice. The reality is that you HAVE to do whatever it is that you are doing, so why not rally up some enthusiasm. There is evidence to support that when you "act" excited, your body chemistry will respond in kind and you will feel better. (I have no idea where this evidence came from. Look it up yourself when you get bored.).

Don't expect everything to be a riveting experience just because you're sober. If that's what you've been told or that's what you're expecting, you'll rapidly be disappointed and become disenchanted with sobriety. Life is not a carnival, unless of course you work at a carnival – and then I'm sure you have bigger life issues than just alcoholism.

Summary: Ultimately, the theme of this chapter is for you to accept the reality that you no longer drink. You don't have to accept (or constantly remind yourself) that you are a weak, powerless or hopeless eternal alcoholic, riddled with flaws and defects. You can if you want to – but why would anyone want to speak about themselves in those terms, especially if you've already turned your life around or are working on it? I'm not going to live in the land of make-believe, but I'm certainly not going to belittle and berate myself. I must simply accept the reality that I no longer drink and I must accept many of the realities that come with being a Re-Invented Alcoholic. I have to approach, appreciate and control my life without the crutch of alcohol.

Reality Worksheet:

What realities listed here must I personally face?: _____

_____

_____

What other realities do I have that weren't listed here?: _____

_____

_____

How can I make the best of these realities?: _____

_____

_____

What realities am I avoiding?: _____

What can I do to better understand my realities?: _____

_____

What actions will I take to deal with my realities?: _____

_____

_____

What behaviors can I get better at so I can accept and control my

realities?: _____

_____

_____

#2) What do YOU want out of sobriety?

"When you don't know what you want you are susceptible to accept anything that comes your way." – Mark A. Tuschel

So I want to ask you, "What do *YOU* want out of sobriety?" I had never been asked this question at a meeting. It was never discussed. It doesn't seem to fall in with any of the traditional 12-steps. Sure, your sponsor may tell you, "If you work the steps the steps will work and you'll regain things that you have lost." But to me that's giving someone false hope and it's far too vague. You need to know and see – in concrete terminology and form – **exactly** what you want to gain, regain, have or do. None of the steps ask you to do this. So I would like you to humor me. I would like you to write out **exactly** what you *want* and *don't want* out of sobriety. Knowing what you *don't want* is equally as important as knowing what you *do want*. In fact, knowing what you don't want may actually be more important to some of you. It's worth the effort to make both lists. I'll be giving you examples of actual lists shortly.

"What you *want* out of sobriety" and "What you *don't want* out of sobriety" are completely selfish questions and they will be the most important questions you will ask yourself in your Re-Invention. Once you have answered these questions in detail, you then have the *core* of what you will do after sobering up. It will also make staying sober a bit easier; in fact, it may make it fun.

The previous sentence might come as a surprise to you, because as you may have already guessed, I am a hardened realist. I offer *no* false hopes that this is going to be either easy or fun. But when you know what you want, you have direction. You will establish values, desires and principles to fall back on when you are tempted to drink. *When you don't know what you want you are susceptible to accept anything that comes your way.*

Doing this written exercise is a great way to eat up sober time. It's also a great way to discover what things are important to you in life. While going through this writing process, you might put down some things you *think* you always wanted in life. As you analyze this particular *want* and consider what needs to be done to accomplish it, you might discover that it's a *want* you truly don't care about or that it was just a fanciful, drunken wish.

Is this tedious, time consuming and mentally taxing? Yes. You're going to have to really think and be introspective. You'll have to think about yourself and about the other people in your life. If you have a spouse or children, you will have to take them into consideration. If you have debts, responsibilities or any other obligations that you're accountable for, you'll have to take them into consideration as well. Is this something that you'll have to do only once? No. Your lists and goals will always be evolving. As you accomplish things on your list, you'll want to continuously update your list because your desires and needs will change as you make progress with your sobriety.

Don't worry whether somebody else sees these titles and lists. "Oh, I don't want anybody to know I'm a drunk." Believe me; I'm sure they already know. And besides, you should be proud to let other people see your lists and for them to see that you want to better your life and that you take this seriously enough to construct a plan. Who knows, when somebody sees your list they may want to help you accomplish your plan, and they'll also probably be a little bit jealous because you've got your shit together enough to know what you want out of life.

As you undertake this exercise, your enthusiasm will increase because you're thinking that everything will now finally start taking shape and things will work out in your life. Here's where I need to remind you that you might not get everything you want out of sobriety. I'm not trying to be a downer or sound depressing. The reality is that some things that you want out of sobriety won't happen. You will get a lot of things out of sobriety and learn a lot about yourself and other people, but just because you want something, make an intelligent plan to accomplish it and do all the right activities to make it happen, doesn't mean it will. The best laid plans don't always work out. And if your expectations are too high or unrealistic, you'll be setting yourself up for failure and that can lead to relapse. I want you to make the lists of what you want and don't want out of living sober and I hope you get all that you desire, but you have to accept that everything you desire won't come to fruition.

Your *wants* need to be realistic. That doesn't mean you don't dream big, but you have to consider whether your wants are *feasible* and *probable*. Let me explain feasible and probable in an analogy. Say for example that one of my *wants* would be to marry a super-model. It's only slightly feasible (and *slightly* is being gracious, it's more a remotely slim chance) but it's not very probable. So my realistic want should be: I want to marry a stable, thoughtful and attractive woman. Now that's feasible and probable, but only if I am stable, thoughtful and keep myself in good shape and maintain a clean appearance. Did my explanation make sense? I hope so.

If you're early into your sobriety, then most likely all you want is to just stay sober, and that's great. But eventually you should want more out of this; you should want to reward yourself for all of your self-control. To me, being a Re-Invented alcoholic isn't just "NOT DRINKING", it's a way of living. It's a way of making the best out of your life and rewarding yourself for your self-control and transferring that self-control into *all* areas of your life. Look, if you wanna be sober and miserable, I don't care. And guess what? Neither does anybody else. You're only robbing yourself if you don't make the best out of this.

On the next few pages you'll see some actual examples of these lists. One set is for a married man and the other is for a single woman. For now, I want to explain how to make a list and how to lay out the list of what you want and don't want and give you some samples of goals to get you thinking.

You will construct two separate lists. One will be titled "What I *want* out of sobriety" and the other will be titled "What I *don't want* out of sobriety." On each of your lists you'll make two columns. On the left will be the **goal or desire** and on the right will be a brief description of **what you need to do to make it happen**.

You want concrete statements or goals, followed by a brief description of the activities that you will have to perform to achieve those goals. You'll also want to periodically review your list, track your progress, accomplishments and your success rate. Is this a lot of tedious work? Yes. But *great things in life don't happen by ambiguous efforts and random activities.* They happen due to focused thought, focused effort and concrete plans.

On top of my lists I like to put the date that I created it. Time passes faster than you realize. Suddenly it's been days, weeks and months since you created your list. When you suddenly look back at it you'll be surprised at how much you've accomplished. It can also be a reminder of what you want or need to do more of. Some things you'll cross off as completed, some you will change to suit your current desires and needs.

You are the only person that knows what you want. Don't be influenced by others telling you what you *should* want. Here are a few sample goals to get you thinking: I want to spend more quality time with my kids, spouse, boyfriend or girlfriend, relatives, family, friends, whoever is important to you in your life. I want to read 20 books this year. I want to save up money for a new car. I want to further my education and get a new job. I want to get a second job. I want to go on a vacation to Florida or wherever. I want to move into a larger or smaller apartment. I want to pay off my mortgage or save enough for a down payment on a house. I want to start an IRA. I want to save a certain amount of money every month towards my retirement. I want to be involved in a certain hobby or a group sport. I want to learn to play the guitar. I want to reach a certain weight – whatever.

Now let me give you some examples for your DON'T want list: I don't want to always be tired and feeling like shit – I do this by staying sober. I don't want to be involved in stupid chaos and other people's drama. I don't want to be the cause of other people's problems. I don't want to always be in debt or constantly increasing it. I don't want to spend money on useless things or things that I can't afford. Again, these are just samples to get you thinking.

The following are actual examples of both lists. One set is from a married man and the other set is from a single woman. I've also included blank outlines for your use. But why not construct your own on a big note pad? There are a variety of styles you can use to make your lists. Try different ones and see which one works best for you.

What I *WANT* out of sobriety

Goals & Desires:	Actions that are needed:
I want to lose 20 pounds and stay at 150 pounds	I do this by going to the gym 3 days a week (M/W/F) I will make sure that I eat a small breakfast, a larger lunch and smaller dinner (after I get done exercising). I will not snack on junk food at night.
I want to save $1,500.00 for a vacation	I do this by by putting $50.00 per week into my "Vacation" passbook savings account. This is less than I normally spent on drinking and I will save by not buying junk food. I will have this automatically withdrawn from my paycheck or I will deposit it at the bank every Monday on my way to the gym. In less than 1 year (30 wks) I will have this vacation money.
I want to spend more time with my kids	I will talk with the kids during dinner. I will dedicate at least 1 hour a night helping and working on their homework with them. I will dedicate my Saturday afternoons to playing with them at home, going to a park or watching them play sports. I want them to know that I'm interested in them.
I want to be a better husband and rebuild our marriage.	I will spend more time with Karen. I will talk with her after the kids go to bed. I will turn off the TV and pay attention to her. I will take Karen on a vacation with the money I have saved. We will decide together on a vacation spot. I will offer to help with some of Karen's chores and I will ask her to help me with some of mine.
I want to get closer to Karen and get along better.	I will talk with Karen during breakfast. I will call her at least once during the day and ask how her day is going. I will pay attention to what she is saying. I will make sure that I say at least one nice thing to her every day. I will ask her what she would like. I will be more romantic and not expect sex in return.

What I *DON'T WANT* out of sobriety

Goals & Desires: | Actions that are needed:

Goals & Desires	Actions that are needed
I don't want to always be late or running behind.	I need to plan ahead better and allow myself more time to get to appointments.
I don't want to wonder about what I said or did the night before.	This is simple. As long as I don't drink, I won't say stupid things or do stupid things that I don't remember.
I don't want to always be apologizing to Karen.	If I don't drink I won't say mean and stupid things to Karen. If I do say something mean, I will apologize for it.
I don't want Karen to have to lie to the kids about where I am or why I can't make it to their game.	As long as I stay sober, I'll be able to spend more time with the kids. I won't be nursing a hangover. If I can't make it to a game or event with the kids I will tell them why.
I don't want to keep getting further in debt.	I will wait 3 days before I make any big purchases. If I want to make a big purchase I will talk with Karen about it. I will charge less and buy less. I will pay an extra $20.00 a month towards credit card debt. After the cards are paid off, I will send an extra $50.00 a month towards the car payment.

Strengths: | Weaknesses:

Strengths	Weaknesses
I know when to keep my mouth shut. I know that debt isn't good for us. I don't like how I feel when I lie.	I give in too easily to impulse purchases. I waste money on dumb stuff when I drink. I'm too easily persuaded by my drinking buddies.

What I *WANT* out of sobriety

Goals & Desires:

Actions that are needed:

Goals & Desires	Actions that are needed
I want to lose 10 pounds and stay at 125 pounds	I will make sure that I exercise at least 3 days a week. I will run or do Pilates if I can't get to the gym. I will eat a small breakfast and healthier dinners. I will make my own lunches. I will not buy junk food.
I want to get a promotion at work.	I will be more involved at work. I'll make sure that supervisors and bosses know that I'm involved and that I care about the company. I will watch the bulletin board for job openings and apply immediately. I will have an updated resume always ready. If the company will pay for school or special training I will take it.
I want to spend more time with my sister.	I won't wait for my sister to call me. I will call her. I will invite her to fun events or I will just invite her over for dinner at my place. We don't always have to go out and get wild. We can just talk. I will let her know that I am no longer drinking.
I want to meet a nice man.	I will make sure that I always look my best when I go out in public. I will smile and carry my head high. I know that I will NOT meet my true love in a bar, so I need to look all around me. If I see someone interesting I will say "Hi." I will not come off as easy and sleazy. I will spend more time at bookstores, the gym and healthy places.
I want to get a new car.	I must spend less money on useless stuff and save more. I will start a new savings account and put the money that I used to spend on drinking and clubbing into it. Once I have saved $1,000 I can start looking at cars.

Strengths:

I am a good looking woman. I am a dedicated employee. I am funny and other people like me when I'm sober. I am a loving woman. I can be a good partner to a decent man.

Weaknesses:

I complain about my problems more than I should. I don't smile enough. I expect others to call me.

What I *DON'T WANT* out of sobriety

Example for Single Female

Goals & Desires: ## Actions that are needed:

I don't want to be in any abusive relationships.	I will respect myself and my time more. I don't need to have a date to feel complete. I will say "no" when it's not a healthy situation for me. I will spend more time with myself if I must.
I don't want to have drama in my life.	This is simple. I just won't drink and I won't hang out with drunks. They only bring me drama. I need to stay in closer touch with my family and my healthy friends.
I don't want to keep putting myself in dangerous situations.	I will not go out and get drunk and act sleazy around scumbag men. I respect my body. I can have fun and go dancing but I won't hang out with drunk guys. I will NOT meet the love of my life in a bar.
I don't want to keep getting further in debt.	I will wait 3 days before I make any big purchases. Sales can wait. I will charge less and buy less. I will go to resale shops more. I will coordinate my current wardrobe better.

Strengths: ## Weaknesses:

I know what is good and safe for me. I am fashion conscious and I can make any outfit look good. I care about people. I am a good judge of character when 'm sober.	I give in too easily to impulse purchases. I get too excited about sales. I feel that I must have a man in my life to be "complete," even if it's just any man.

What I *WANT* out of sobriety

Date:_____

Goals & Desires: **Actions that are needed:**

Strengths: **Weaknesses:**

What I *DON'T WANT* out of sobriety

Date:_____

Goals & Desires: **Actions that are needed:**

Strengths: **Weaknesses:**

Summary: This will be a writing task that you will be doing for the rest of your sober life. So what? If you don't know what you want (and don't want) out of sobriety, you'll never know if you got it. If you're going to go through all the effort to live sober then why not make sobriety work for you?

This exercise alone will help stave off boredom, depression, self-pity, guilt and frustration. Sometimes it's scary to see your life on paper – where you can clearly see your limitations and obstacles. But this is a very POWERFUL exercise. It will remind you that you are serious about sobriety. It will show others that you are serious about sobriety.

Again, these are just some examples to get you thinking on your own. I can't tell you what you want and don't want and neither should anyone else. I can help get you thinking, but these decisions should be your own. When you make decisions on your own, you become responsible for those decisions, and regardless of whether they're good or bad decisions, this will help build your self-esteem. And isn't that what you want? To be proud of yourself, to respect yourself, to hold yourself in high self-esteem? That's what being a Re-Invented alcoholic is all about.

Do yourself a favor that will be a huge benefit to you. Make these two lists, "What I want and what I DON'T want out of living sober." These lists may be the thing that saves you from relapse one day. You're sitting there all depressed feeling sorry for yourself, you're right on the edge, you could easily go out and get all fucked up – but you see your list and it brings you back to why you want to stay sober. Please do this for yourself. If you don't know what you want you'll never know if this is worth the effort.

Wants Worksheet:

Have I made a list of what I want out of sobriety?: _____

Are my wants realistic?: _____

Have I listed the activities of what I must do?: _____

Have I made my *don't want* list?: _____

Have I placed this list in plain view so I can see it daily?: _____

Have I discussed my wants with the important people in my life who

may be involved or helpful?: _____

How often will I update or check my list to see what I have

accomplished?: _____

#3) Develop a reward system

"Alcoholics will admit to anything except how much money they spend on booze." – Mark A. Tuschel

Human behavior is driven by the desire for pleasure (a reward) or the avoidance of pain. You might question this statement. "I hated myself for drinking. I had plenty of pain because of it. So why did I keep doing it?" Because your immediate pleasure reward was catching a buzz or getting outright drunk. The pain came afterward as a consequence of that immediate reward. Then the pain and problems became protracted, they intensified, and the only way to avoid the pain was to go for the immediate pleasure of getting drunk again. The cycle of self-destruction was now in place.

As a sober person, you want to allow those natural human drives – desire for pleasure and the avoidance of pain – to work for you in a constructive way. So you need to reward yourself, but the rewards will be delayed and by using your self-control the pain will be avoided.

The reason for rewarding yourself is to experience a concrete benefit for your self-control. The elimination of problems, drama, debt and bad occurrences can be a reward in itself, but it isn't always that noticeable. You don't feel rewarded because the lack of bad shit doesn't stand out the same way the occurrence of bad shit will. A tangible reward will stand out more and it will confirm your resolve and validate your decision to live sober.

The anticipation of delayed gratification can be more fun and exhilarating than getting the actual reward itself. For instance, have you ever been excited about going to see a certain movie, taking a vacation, attending a party or seeing someone? Then when it was over you felt, "Well that wasn't that great." The experience may have been pleasant (or maybe not), but it was the *anticipation* that was more exciting than the actual event.

Anticipation can be used to motivate you to stay sober. Looking forward to receiving your reward, letting it distract you and drive your self-control is using anticipation. For instance, "I'm not going to drink today so I can save another $10 towards my vacation." Another example would be, "I had a bad day at work and I feel like drinking, but if I drink I won't be able to get my new car. As long as I stay sober tonight I'll be one day closer to getting my car." Another illustration is, "I'll clean the kitchen, wash the dishes and clear the counters. When it's all done I can sit down and watch a movie." You are controlling your current behavior, feelings and thinking by anticipating something you will enjoy in the future.

You must decide what types of rewards you want and what rewards will motivate you. This is an activity that will require you to think. You should also write out or print up your reward system so you can see it. When you can see it in front of you, you will have a higher probability of following your plan. You will then have to exhibit self-control and stick to your plan. A big part of sticking to your plan is to make sure that you enjoy your rewards, but only after you have exhibited the behavior to earn them.

With this in mind, I believe that you should devise a multi-tiered reward system. This means having some immediate rewards in place for you to enjoy daily, some midrange rewards and long-term rewards. Following is an example of a multi-tiered reward schedule. I'm also including examples of rewards, but these are just ideas. You have to decide what rewards you desire.

- **Daily rewards for daily accomplishments:** Treat yourself to a small amount of some self-indulgent snack. Watch a certain TV show or watch a DVD for a specified amount of time. Call friends or relatives to chat on the phone (starting at a specified time). Just sit and relax.

- **Weekly rewards:** Special meal, special cut of meat or some other luxurious food. Coffee at Starbucks on Sunday mornings. Buy a magazine. Rent a movie and watch it. Book(s). Music from iTunes.

- **Monthly rewards:** Go out to see a movie. Go out to dinner with your spouse or friend(s). Go to an event with your kids (amusement park, beach, fair or festival, movie).

- **Annual rewards:** Holiday gifts. Birthday gifts. Vacation. Home furnishings (furniture, new TV, new mattress, whatever.) Personal items (new cell phone, electronic gadget, etc.)

- **Long-term rewards:** A new car, boat, camper, down payment on a house.

Does all this sound like sacrifice and being a control freak? Probably. But without control, shit gets out of hand and the best laid plans go awry. Without self-control and a bit of sacrifice, rewards mean nothing. You are sacrificing destructive and nonproductive activity for constructive and rewarding results.

Use your specifically saved *booze money* to purchase these reward items (I'll talk about savings accounts shortly). Consciously say to yourself, while you're shopping or paying, "This is my reward. I saved this money by not drinking. I can afford it and I deserve it as a reward for my self-control."

What do you think is the one thing most drinkers hate to admit or don't want to talk about? Go ahead and think I'll give you a few seconds. Okay, times up. We'll openly admit to being an alcoholic, we'll say that we're powerless over alcohol, we'll hand our authority over to a higher power, we'll go apologize to the world, make amends to everyone we've ever known and spread the good word of sobriety – but we'll do anything to avoid sitting down with a pen and a pad of paper and do a realistic accounting of what our drinking has cost us in terms of actual money. That's because it's personal, the numbers really hit home.

People will often complain that they're always broke, they can't make ends meet, they don't make enough money, they don't get paid enough. Bullshit! I'm poor and I can make ends meet. I have had to accept that I must live within my means. I can't buy (or worse yet – charge) everything I want. I have to cut expenses and forgo some things. Look, if you can afford all the costs associated with drinking, what do I care what you do with your money. But most of us barely make enough to cover our bills and save some money for the future. But making ends meet, living within your means and saving money can be done.

I have talked with a lot of former drunks who say, "I've saved thousands of dollars since I quit drinking." My question then is: "How much? Where is it?" Their only response is that they've saved thousands. If you don't have a concrete method of tracking how much you've saved, you'll never get to enjoy the reward. You'll even think that you've saved more than you actually have. But you still don't have it unless you put it away somewhere.

My financial situation turned around the very next day after I quit drinking. No, all my bills didn't magically disappear – but I wasn't literally pissing money away anymore and I immediately began paying off my debt. It went from paying off debt, to paying off my car to paying off my home and then to saving and investing money. Hey, I'm a shit-fer-brains, and if I can do it YOU can do it.

A simple way to save money and enjoy it more is to not spend your hard earned money on getting drunk. So if you no longer spend money on beer, wine, liquor, at bars and clubs, what do you do with it? How about starting a savings account? I can't stress enough the importance and value of stashing away money that you had once been spending on booze. If you don't stash it away, it will end up being spent on something else by default and you'll never see or feel the concrete reward of what you're saving.

Money is a universally accepted means of reward (so is sex but I'll just stick with money here). You may have other intangible rewards that are of more importance to you than money. I'll get to those shortly, but money can be a way for you to get some of those intangibles.

I like it when people say, "money isn't everything." My response: "You're right, money isn't everything... it's the only fucking thing!" Before you write me off as money grubbing and evil, please continue reading.

You don't need tons of money, but who's kidding who? Without money you can't eat, pay your bills, live well, afford your family or children all of the comforts that you would like them to have and enjoy. Without money you are stressed, tensions build and you're not able to enjoy simple pleasures in life – because the stress of being broke or in debt is continually haunting. The GREED of money is BAD. To earn money is GOOD. To earn a decent living through your own ethical work and effort is GOOD. Money isn't bad, greed is bad. Be proud of yourself; never feel the need to apologize for earning a decent living that's a result of your own hard work and effort.

Is it plagiarism if I steal from myself? I don't believe that it is, so I'm going to use some ideas and a few excerpts from my other book; *Living Sober Sucks (but living drunk sucks more)*. Chapter #13 – Mark's Reward System. Some of the material that you'll read has already been stated, but it's so important that I believe it's worth repeating.

> **Start a Savings Account:** I suggest that you start a separate *Sobriety Savings Account*. This should be a ***Passbook Savings Account***. The reason I want you to start a Passbook account is because you physically have to take the Passbook to the bank to withdraw money. You can't simply access or withdraw money online. Physically having to go to the bank will give you time to think whether you really need to take this money out or not and you won't be so easily tempted to impulsively spend it. As I've mentioned, you could always come up with money for

> drinking, so for every day that you don't drink, put $10.00 into this savings account. You know that you spent at least $10.00 a day on drinking. So instead of stopping at the bar every day on your way home from work, stop at the bank and deposit $10.00 into a savings account. Yes - do it every day! The bank doesn't care how much or how often you deposit money, that's what they're there for. The reason that I suggest you make a deposit every day is twofold: First, you want to make it a habit, and second, if you let that money pile up on your dresser that fifty bucks looks real tempting at the end of the week – you might end up spending it on something foolish. Do this for one month and you'll have $300.00. Stay sober for 90 days and you'll have accumulated $900.00 and after one year you will have saved up over $3,600.00.

I personally like the old-school system of cashing my paycheck. I deposit what I need to cover bills then I get some cash back for daily expenses. No debit cards. That way I know where my money is going and it makes me think twice about impulsive and small purchases. I also like the act of taking what would have been my drinking money (cash) and depositing it into my *sobriety savings account*. I can see the balance grow (immediate reward) and I'm practicing self-discipline. Eventually I withdraw some money to reward myself, to buy Christmas gifts, whatever (delayed gratification).

Just like your *wants* and *don't wants* from Chapter #2, your rewards must be realistic, both probable and feasible. For instance, let's say you want to reward yourself with a new car. You decide that you want the reward of a brand new BMW M-6 convertible. That's a $120,000.00 car! Is it feasible? Sure, if you save $20 a day for the next 16-½ years. And in 16-½ years that car will cost even more. So is this probable? No.

So let's look at what *is* both probable and feasible. You likely spent a conservative average of $10 a day on drinking (I'll explain how I arrived at this figure shortly). By putting $10 a day into a *sobriety savings account*, you'll have $3,650.00 after one year. That's enough for a down payment on a really nice new or used car. Let me take this a step further. If the car cost a total of $20,000.00 (with tax, title, etc.) and you put down $3,650.00, your continued $10 a day *sobriety savings* would almost cover the monthly payments (based on a 4 year loan). This is a realistic reward.

How did I arrive at this $10 average? You say you didn't drink every day. Humor me here and play along. Let's say you'd go out on Friday night and spend $40 at a bar (don't forget to add in smokes, cover charge, bar gambling games and food afterwards). On Saturday you go to a concert or music club and you spend another $40 (don't forget to count pot or any other recreational drug you might have also bought). On Sunday you have a couple beers or some wine at home to take the edge off. Maybe you went out to a nice restaurant and your bar bill is $60. Or you entertained at home and supplied your guests with beer, wine and liquor. Hosting parties and drinking at home costs a lot of money as well.

So realistically, you probably spent $100 (or more) over the weekend. Divide $100 by 7 days and you average $14.28 per day. Let's say you were to put that money into savings instead. That comes to $428.57 a month. Think that would make your car payment? Think that would help pay your rent or pay down your mortgage? How about you do that for 3 months, that comes to $1,285.71. Would that pay for a nice vacation? Or a new TV or something nice for your family or kids?

Conservatively, you probably spent at least $10 a day, on average, for your drinking hobby. So you should put at least $10 a day into your *sobriety savings* account. You don't have a sobriety savings account? Then start one.

Here is another brief excerpt from: *Living Sober Sucks.*

> **It isn't just money that helps me enjoy my sober life:** Positively based rewards don't have to be exclusively materialistic. Think about the loving relationships you can rebuild. The friendships that will grow deeper. The clarity of your own thoughts. The personal pride and higher self-esteem you will feel. How much healthier you will be. Think about the great sex you will be able to have while sober.
>
> Now that I am sober, I find that I use my mind and my time far more efficiently. I enjoy my work and my projects more. I reward myself by spending more time playing with

my dogs. I spend more time working in my yard and making my house look nice. I spend more time helping friends with their home projects and I spend more time having deeper relationships with my friends. I go to a gym to exercise, which rewards me with better health and higher levels of self-esteem. I read a lot of books to further my knowledge. I stay very busy doing things for me, my family and my friends. And when I'm just sitting around *fuckin' off*, I don't feel guilty - I can truly relax.

I urge you to do some math homework and figure out what you used to spend on drinking. I've had some people tell me how depressed they got after realizing how much they wasted in their life on booze and drugs. Look, that money is gone, never to be seen again. Don't hate yourself for it – you can't get THAT money back. But what you can do is learn to start stashing away some of that money you no longer spend on booze and drugs.

I'm not lecturing you; I was guilty of this shit myself. I didn't want to admit what drinking cost me. But once I did figure it out, I realized that I could be doing a lot more for myself with that money than just getting drunk. It's your money, do what you want with it, put it into savings, start a mutual fund account or spend it on frivolous things. Now that you've quit drinking, why not let that drinking money work for you and let sobriety reward you, with less debt and a few nice things in life.

Summary: Life is not meant to be all sacrifice and suffering. You will sacrifice destructive, immediate gratification so you can enjoy future rewards. You should indulge yourself with some type of pleasurable rewards: short-term, monthly, annual and long-term. Problems arise when you compare your life to someone else's life or to their values and reward system. You can desire and aspire to achieve what others have, but comparing your life to someone else's will only arouse feelings of inadequacy within you. Your rewards should be realistic to your financial condition, meaning feasible and probable.

You must have a detailed plan. Without a plan you are susceptible to acting and reacting on impulses. It is very important that you reward yourself in some fashion according to your plan. Without concrete rewards you will not see any evidence of your efforts and staying sober will feel unrewarding. All rewards don't have to be materialistic. Your reward could be spending more time with people or your pets. Exercising more, cooking more, reading more or simply relaxing and doing nothing. Be proud of yourself, enjoy your rewards and remind yourself that you have earned these rewards.

Reward Worksheet:

Have I started a *sobriety savings account*?: _____

Short term savings goal (30 days): _____

How much to stash away per day: _____

This is what I want to buy at the end of 30 days: _____

This is what I want to buy at the end of 90 days: _____

_____

This is what I want to buy at the end of 1 year: _____

_____

These are the *things* I eventually want to buy with my sobriety savings:

_____

_____

This is how much money I need to save every day to afford these things:

_____

These are the *intangible rewards* I want to enjoy: _____

_____

_____

#4) Further your mind

"Knowledge is power, but it's not <u>powerful</u> until you use it."
Mark A. Tuschel.

You're reading *this* book, so once you're done with it, start reading another book. It doesn't matter what the subject matter or the genre is, just keep reading. In fact, I believe that you should read about subjects that you're unfamiliar with. You might discover a new passion or interest. The mission is to challenge your mind, to cause you to think, to learn new perspectives and to learn new things.

Reading and learning will give you something to do during those periods of boredom. As you expand your knowledge you might discover new hobbies or things that interest you. For instance, while reading a magazine you discover that there's a large market for vintage and antique fishing lures. You happen to be familiar with lures because your grandfather used to take you fishing. As you do more research, you learn how to set up an eBay account. Then you find yourself going to yard sales on weekends looking to buy old fishing gear. You know exactly what to look for and how to resell it on eBay. Suddenly you have a hobby that involves your mind, keeps you busy and might earn you a few extra dollars. I'm using fishing lures as an example. Who knows what you will find interesting when you begin to expand your knowledge.

Another way to consume boring times is to go to bookstores. You can walk into any bookstore and spend hours browsing and paging through books. Walk around and see if any sections draw you in. A good area for Re-Invented Alcoholics is the self-help section, you'll find a myriad of books about a variety of subjects. Walk over to the psychology and philosophy section and start browsing. Reading books on psychology and human behavior will help you understand yourself better, which will ultimately help you make the best out of living sober.

Make it a point to read different genres of books. If you've never read fiction or novels, read a couple of them. You don't know what topics or authors you might find interesting. Read magazines and publications about hobbies or sports that you have interest in. Just read. You'll be shocked at how you interpret reading and what you can learn with a sober mind.

The most important book to have in your library is the dictionary. The more you read the more new words you will encounter. Some authors are excellent at using an expansive vocabulary. The context in which they use their vibrant vocabulary almost explains a given word's meaning. Don't automatically assume that you know the meaning of an unfamiliar word. When you encounter a new word, look it up in your dictionary. You'll then understand how the author intended to use it and you'll learn alternative meanings of the word. I might sound like a nerd, but this word learning process *can* be exciting.

When you are knowledgeable on a variety of subjects and have expanded your own vocabulary, conversations will become deeper and more engaging. When you acquire knowledge of a subject you will be able to support your own position and opinion better; far better than drunkenly saying, "Fuck you, you don't know shit." You may still respond to someone with those words, but at the very least you'll be able to follow up with an intelligent explanation of why you think the other person doesn't know shit.

Sober conversations can be very stimulating. They bring a higher level of closeness between you and the other person. This is not to say that all conversations will be with friends or loved ones. These conversations can occur among people with whom you vehemently disagree, but it enables exchange and respect for one another. Sure, drunken conversations may have also been stimulating and intimate; through the telling of secrets, agreeing with one another and gossiping about others. But these were just drunken conversations which probably had little substance behind them. And as I'm sure we have all experienced, those drunken conversations can turn awfully ugly in a flash.

Sober discussions will lead to more profound thoughts and connections with other people. This can be a launch pad for you to do some follow-up research on the topic discussed and re-engage the conversation at a future point. You have no idea what you might learn from the other person, and you have no idea what you might learn by doing research to support your own opinion.

Expansion of knowledge and vocabulary exposes you to the world and to more options. It also opens up your mind to understanding alternative and opposite views. Being able to understand alternative and differing views will allow you to better accept other people's behavior and allow you the ability to embrace sober reality better. This doesn't mean that you have to agree with everyone's opinions and beliefs. It will actually protect you from falling prey to unhealthy and destructive influences. Having correct knowledge and being able to support your opinions intelligently will result in higher self-esteem and help you stay faithful to your personal beliefs, morals and principles.

Reading isn't the only way of exercising your mind. The act of writing requires thought and introspection. For example, my writing of this book requires me to think, organize my thoughts, choose words, look up words and study the craft of writing. You can do the same by starting your own blog, journaling or creating a diary. Your writing doesn't have to be about you or your alcohol issues. You can try your hand at writing stories, mysteries, sci-fi, erotica, whatever you desire.

At this point I'd like to cite a real-life example about blogging. Sara Mcdaniels contacted me via email through my website, www.LivingSoberSucks.com Sara is a single mother with three children. We began emailing back and forth discussing sobriety. Sara felt she had some hidden urge within her to write, but she had never done it before. She asked me a simple question, "How do you write?" I told her that all you do is just start writing, "Say what's in your heart. Write for yourself and don't worry if you don't think it's any good. Just write."

Sara embarked on educating herself about blogging and webpage design. She then began organizing her thoughts. A month later she had created a very polished looking blog site for single mothers. www.complicatedlifeofasinglemon.blogspot.com Sara challenged her mind and then went and did what she wanted to do. Her fan base has grown and this has become a mentally and emotionally rewarding activity for her. It has evolved into an interactive site for other single mothers to post comments, share stories and ask questions. Sara is a great example of what someone can do with their mind when they challenge it and take action. You never know what *you* can do until you at least try.

Interacting with posts on all the various social medias will get you writing as well. Don't just tweet, "I farted," actually write something of interest and engage in intelligent banter. Virtually every website or article online has a place for you to post a comment. Express your opinions and get involved by posting your own commentaries. You can spend more time writing deeper, detailed emails to friends and family. You could even go to the extent of hand writing letters and cards to friends. When writing on your computer, please enable your spell check or run your writing through a spell checker before sending or posting. Why? Because you will learn new words, the correct spelling, definition and usage of words.

Writing isn't just mentally stimulating, it challenges your mind and it requires thought. You have to take the thoughts that are in your mind, convert those thoughts into written form, then convey those same thoughts, mental images and messages into the mind of the reader. This will require you to think imaginatively and creatively. You'll have to think things through in greater detail. And don't make excuses like, "I'm not really good at writing." It's coming from *you* and that's what makes it special. With practice you will get better at it.

Just because you graduated from high school or college doesn't mean that you stop learning. I never graduated from high school (I thought I was too smart for school and I entered the working world), but I eventually continued my education in the Air Force and on my own. You don't have to be involved in some sort of formal, accredited schooling. You can attend classes on subjects just because you like them. It could be night classes, online classes or community colleges in your area. There may be continuing education that's offered through your workplace. There could be seminars and extra training courses as well. If you're so compelled, you could return to school fulltime with the intention of acquiring a degree and then pursuing a new career.

Another mentally stimulating activity that's often overlooked is volunteering. I'm not referring to just volunteering to help at a bake sale or selling raffle tickets for your church; I'm talking about volunteering for causes that involve deeper thought. You could volunteer to be involved with a political movement, environmental group, animal shelter, social or religious organization. There are discussion groups which gather regarding these subjects as well. The idea is for you to get involved with something that requires you to think, talk and interact with other people.

There are intellectually challenging hobbies that you can do alone. Crossword puzzles, shape puzzles, old-fashioned jigsaw puzzles, Sudoku puzzles or mentally challenging board games. You might be thinking, "Oh c'mon Mark. This is silly. Board games and puzzles aren't exciting. I want excitement!" Well sorry, mental stimulation isn't ever going to offer the same type of short-term excitement as getting drunk will. Use your mental creativity to turn a simple board game into some excitement. Try playing "Strip Scrabble" sometime – now that's exciting and arousing.

I agree that getting drunk can be mentally challenging. You have to think about walking straight and talking straight. You have to think about where you are, what you're saying, what you're doing. That's challenging, but not in a constructive way. Conversely, getting drunk is not mentally stimulating. It's actually biochemically numbing to your brain which then makes it even more difficult to think. As a drunk you had to really focus your mind at times and use it in many creative ways. "How will I get home? Where is my home? How can I get there without being arrested for drunk driving? How will I explain this? How can I pay for this?" The list could go on. Now that you're sober use that same mental focus and creativity to further your mind.

Sobriety in and of itself doesn't automatically make you smarter or increase your knowledge. Nor does it guarantee that all your thoughts and decisions will be correct. You will need to constantly be learning new knowledge, checking your premises and correcting your errors. Like Sara, it is up to you to challenge your mind, to take action and to make your mind work for you. You will have to feed your own mind with knowledge and then exercise it.

Summary: Mental stimulation and mental challenges are a completely different type of excitement and arousal than getting drunk. Engage and challenge your mind. Ask questions, not just of others but of yourself as well. Invest time in expanding your knowledge and furthering your education. Let your curiosity get the best of you. Read, perform research, write and interact with other minds.

It isn't necessary to possess a high I.Q. to challenge your mind. Regardless of your own personal learning capabilities and mental capacity, you can always further your knowledge. Raw intellect and formal education does not make someone wise. Knowledge, experience and the proper use of knowledge is what makes someone wise. Being able to support your opinions intelligently by possessing correct knowledge will result in higher feelings of self-esteem and help you stay faithful to your personal beliefs, morals and principles.

Further your mind Worksheet:

How can I challenge my mind?: _____

_____

_____

What types of books would I like to read?: _____

_____

_____

What activities are mentally stimulating for me?: _____

_____

_____

What type of entertainment is mentally stimulating for me?: _____

_____

_____

How will I use my mind to make my life better?: _____

_____

_____

What subjects or topics would I like to have more knowledge of?: _____

_____

_____

How will I use all of the new knowledge I am learning?: _____

_____

_____

always loved playing basketball behind the garage with my dad.

Team and group sports can also elevate your competitive nature. This can be a positive thing. When you have the desire to be a more competitive opponent, you'll need to improve your skills and you will undoubtedly spend more time practicing. This results in you spending more time exercising. So this works in your favor; you exercise more, burn up aggressions and do something with sober bored time. Sports and physical hobbies are a lot more enjoyable when you are stronger and when your muscle development is structured around participating in a given sport.

Every physical sport or hobby isn't bodily demanding. If you golf, you can walk the course instead of using a cart and carry or pull your bag. Hiking and hunting can be done alone. Gardening and general yard work can require a fair amount of exertion. Take your dog for walks. If you don't have a dog, ask a neighbor or a friend if you can walk theirs, or just go with them when they walk their dog. Woodworking, sewing, playing the guitar or piano requires physical dexterity and eye-hand control. The physical actions require mental focus.

These are just a few ideas. You need to discover what you would like to do. There are plenty of hobbies and sports that don't require extreme physical exertion but will still keep your body moving, the blood pumping and your mind sharp.

Diet: As long as you're not drinking why not eat healthier? You'll have more money available to buy good food that you enjoy – so eat well. And if you're exercising or involved in a physically demanding hobby, you'll want to put proper fuel into your body. Eating ice-cream and cake may fill you up, but it won't aid in building the necessary muscles required for strength. Do some research or talk with a dietician to find out what types of foods are most beneficial to support your personal exercise regimen.

If you typically eat fast foods, the same basic meal every day, or have never paid attention to the kinds of food you eat, why not try some new foods? This can be an exciting undertaking for you. Experiment with different recipes and new flavors. Take notice how certain foods might excite your taste buds and how other foods make you feel physically. Do certain foods make you tired? Do some energize you? Which are your favorites? Cooking and experimenting with recipes is another way of using up sober time. You can invite a friend over to be your test dummy. It can be a lot of fun cooking for or with someone. Who knows, you might find cooking to be an exciting new hobby for you.

Some people have been known to gain weight after they quit drinking. This is a result of them sitting around and stuffing their faces with comfort foods, which is an action brought on by boredom or self-pity. Instead of getting fatter, make this an opportunity for you to lose unwanted weight. Just as you are now controlling what you *don't* put into your body (alcohol), pay attention to and control what types and how much food you *do* put into your body. Beer, wine, alcohol and the mixers that go with it are high in empty calories. Drinking is generally done while you're sedentary. So the alcohol goes straight to your brain and the calories go straight to your ass. If you're going to replace alcohol with eating, then make sure that it's healthy, exciting and properly proportioned foods. When you weigh less, you'll feel better, have higher self-esteem and you'll feel more like being physically active.

Summary: Most of what I've talked about here is common sense, but drunks aren't famous for having common sense. Exercise, a healthy diet and food consumption require discipline and self-control. These are areas of your life that you do have total control over. Regardless of your physical conditions or mobility limitations, there are exercises that you can participate in. Being physically fit and maintaining a healthy weight is an outward expression to others that you care about yourself. Being sedentary will only fuel feelings of boredom and self-pity. You will have to force yourself to begin and continue being active. Furthering your body and being in better physical shape will boost your self-esteem.

Further your body Worksheet:

What type of exercises will I do?: _____

_____

_____

How often will I exercise?: _____

_____

What is my goal for exercising?: _____

_____

What physical activities do I like?: _____

_____

_____

What will I do to make sure I am more active and involved in them?:

_____

_____

What hobbies do I like?: _____

_____

_____

What will I do to make sure I am more active and involved in them?:

_____

_____

What new hobbies or activities would I like to try?: _____

_____

_____

#6) Relationships, family and friends

"Sobriety doesn't guarantee shit." – *Anonymous*

Sobriety and relationships are a rusty double-edged sword. The sword cuts alright, but it never cuts clean and the wounds can be ugly and take a long time to heal. The ending of friendships, marriages, relationships and rifts between family members can shatter your heart and last a lifetime. These dissolutions may have come as a result of your past drinking or due to your current sobriety. On the positive side, sobriety will bring you closer together with some friends, relationships and family members.

All interaction that you have with another person can be considered a relationship. As basic or simple as some relationships may seem, they are still complicated because each relationship has its own unique elements. As a sober person, you must re-learn how to deal with all these relationships. A key factor is accepting the other person as they are and accepting yourself as you are. The best scenario is when both you and the other person mutually decide how valuable and desirable the relationship is to one another. Sometimes you will have to make that decision on your own, based upon what's in your best interest for maintaining your sobriety.

The people whom you are in direct contact with play a bigger role in your sobriety than you may care to admit. It would be unrealistic (and poor advice) to boil every type of relationship down into simplistic terms. In this chapter I will be giving you many examples of real scenarios from my own life. I'll offer some ideas for your consideration and present ways in which you can resolve relationship dilemmas. Ultimately you are the only one who will live your life and therefore you will have to make these relationship decisions on your own. Some will be painful, some will be beneficial. You won't always make the right decision. Hopefully this chapter will help you make fewer wrong decisions.

Relationships: You have individual relationships with family members and friends. What I'm going to talk about here are the intimate and romantic relationships that you have with specific people in your life. This refers to your spouse, lover, partner, etc. I'm going to use some excerpts from *Living Sober Sucks*.

> If you are in a marriage or relationship and both of you are alcoholics, try to sober up together. If you do this alone, you may find yourself ALONE. The butt-ugly truth is that if you are the only one living sober, then the two of you will be going in different directions from one another. It is sad and difficult to accept, but you very well might have to leave your relationship. This is not always the case, but living in an alcoholic household while you're trying to lead a sober life doesn't give you much of a chance at success. Sometimes you just have to do what you have to do.

> **Spouse/Partner that drinks:** The renewed relationship with your spouse or partner is predicated on the presumption that they are supportive of you and they are not drinking either. If they drink and have an attitude of, "Look, alcohol is your problem. Why should I quit just because you can't handle it?" Then this is not a healthy position for you to be in and sadly, the relationship probably won't work. Keep in mind that I said *probably*. You can be with a partner that drinks socially, as long as it

doesn't bother or tempt you. They still need to show some respect of your efforts and not drink to excess.

If you demand that your spouse/partner stops drinking because you did, you are setting the stage for arguments and confrontation and they may harbor some ill emotions towards you. They may use this demand against you (unconsciously) as a bargaining tool. You might hear statements like, "I quit drinking for you and you still haven't changed... you don't spend more time with the kids... you don't take me out more... you haven't found a decent job... etc." The list could go on. You might even find yourself saying these things to your spouse after you have quit. Using statements like this and arguing will not help control your temptations to drink. Drinking again will not be a way of getting back at your partner, it will only harm you. Your spouse/partner needs to be *willing* to stop drinking with you and because they *want* to support you.

I want to stop drinking but my spouse, partner doesn't want to. Naturally, it's best if you both work on this together and help support each other. Your partner might not feel that they have a problem or simply doesn't want to stop. If you are married or in a committed relationship, it isn't unreasonable to ask your partner to abstain with you. If they cooperate, but do it grudgingly, this may cause more friction. If your partner willingly stops drinking with you, you then have an obligation to show them your gratitude. You need to thank them and learn to show them your appreciation for their help. This doesn't give them a license to abuse, mistreat or take advantage of you. Ultimately you have to focus on your own sobriety. With that said, it may be in your best interest to get out of the relationship if your spouse doesn't want to stop drinking. I would never want to be instrumental in advising someone to needlessly end a

have a responsibility to work as a team. It will require patience, compassion, flexibility and effort on your behalf. You will have to spend more time together maybe even go to counseling together. You can expect a few snags and difficulties as you work on this together. It may not work out as you hoped or planned but you have clearly made progress if the other person is willing to try.

No guarantees here: I do not guarantee that ultimatums will work. I do not guarantee that talking with someone about their alcohol problem will have any positive effect. Alcohol is an inanimate enemy that completely takes command over an alcoholics' mind when in their system. Nothing will change until the alcoholic is willing to exert self-control and willpower to keep alcohol out of their system. The best advice I can pass along is to just keep trying. Keep offering your help, keep doing something. You have to believe that at some point a breakthrough will occur. I realize how simplistic and hokey that statement sounds, but other than totally giving up on a person and walking away, what alternative is there?

Even as I live sober, I still make some incorrect relationship decisions. I have ended romantic relationships in error. The other person in the romantic relationship was a social drinker, and I as a sober person decided that this wasn't a good or safe environment for me to be in. What did I do wrong? I didn't ask or make the request that they stop drinking. I did the thinking for the other person. I allowed *myself* to believe that the other person would make certain decisions and I didn't allow *them* the opportunity to make their own decisions. You don't know what you don't know. You need to ask the other person questions if you are unsure of something or if the decision involves another person. Just because you ask doesn't mean that the other person will give you the answer that you're hoping for or that they won't lie. People do lie or are unsure themselves. Asking and conversing will at least give the other person an opportunity to express their point of view before you needlessly end a friendship, marriage or relationship.

Family: "You can pick your friends but you can't pick your family." That's true, but you can decide how much time you spend with your family. Before I get too far into this subject, I wish to acknowledge that every situation is different. You may be obligated or required to spend time with family members who are destructive towards your sobriety. Certain living conditions and family structures are completely out of your control – kind of. There are some things that *are* within your control, namely your actions and reactions. I know, easier said than done.

I fully understand that family dynamics and conditions are not always the best or what you would like them to be. I deal with some family conditions and responsibilities that I did not ask for nor want. If it weren't for the fact that these people are "blood," I would have nothing to do with them. In this situation, I have established boundaries upon myself. I will only allow myself to be drawn into their problems so far. I will fulfill the duties and obligations that I have agreed upon or am legally responsible for and no more. I have learned from experience that I can ache over someone's plight, offer my help and assistance, be responsible for them, do all their work for them – only to be let down. This is why I have established personal boundaries for myself, in order to preserve my own sanity and life. Sacrificing my own time, health or life will not help my family members.

Some families are all drunks and getting hammered is the accepted norm. Some families aren't necessarily a bunch of drunks but drinking is part of their social behavior. These types of environments could be where your drinking roots stem from. Now that you no longer drink, you can accept your family's drinking habits and control your own behavior or avoid getting together

79

with your family. I'm sure that you know people who agonize over going to family gatherings. "All they do is get drunk and argue. My brother gets blasted and passes out, my dad gets belligerent and my sister starts crying. I hate it." That might be *your* situation. If that's the case, all you can do is attend and do your best to not engage. It sucks but sometimes that's just the way it is.

When I talk about family I'm not only referring to your blood relatives. This can include extended family and in-laws. For example, my family (and former in-laws) would come over to my house for birthdays, holidays, parties, whatever. If I got drunk and annoying then they would leave. I never noticed this because I was drunk. And yes, I've had to call friends and family members the next day and apologize for my behavior. But ultimately what they were doing was protecting themselves by leaving. Not protection against physical harm by me, but protecting themselves against my boisterous drunkenness. They didn't want to listen to my shit so they left. You may have to do the same. Make your obligatory appearance and get the hell out of there as soon as you can.

Conversely, your family might be overjoyed that you no longer drink. My family is an example. Now that I'm sober we spend more time together. They stay longer for gatherings and we actually enjoy the events more. The food is better and we all engage in conversation, no one is avoiding me. I'm not inferring that it's all warm and fuzzy joy. We're family; so we insult one another, crack jokes and argue, but it's not drunken, belligerent behavior. I have gotten much closer with my family members. I don't avoid them and they don't avoid me. We have actually become very good friends. My sobriety has in fact created a tighter bond within our family.

I have not included children in this discussion because your children *are* your responsibility. Like it or not, you have an obligation to them; morally and legally. You may have to make some sacrifices for the wellbeing of your children. But remember that if you are unfit, unhealthy, stressed out and tapped out, you won't be of any use to them whatsoever.

Friendships: Many of my past friendships have ended as a result of my sober lifestyle. But for every friend that I've lost I've gained two new ones and the friends who've remained have become more valuable to me. If I don't pay close attention and do an accounting of my friends, I would never see how beneficial this has been.

Losses, be they financial or friendships, seem to stand out more in the memory than gains do. If I only remember and think about the friends that I've lost, that would be disrespectful and a disservice to my current friends. Keep this in mind the next time you call someone and say, "This sobriety sucks. I'm lonely, I don't have any friends and I have no one to hang out with or talk to." Don't laugh; I've been on the receiving end of phone calls like that. When the person said that to me it made me think, "Well what am I? A nobody? You're talking to me. Don't I count as a friend?"

You might have to tell some of your old, long lost acquaintances that you no longer drink. This might help rekindle your friendship with them and you won't have to go searching for new friends. A key element with friendships is that you also have to be a good friend in return. Ask yourself objective questions: Would I want to hang out with me? Am I fun to be around or am I always whining and complaining? Do I *expect* people to be my friend? Do I put *conditions* on my friendship? Is this particular friendship helpful towards my continued sobriety?

Some of your friendships will come to an end. Many of my friendships ended simply because I no longer drink, but those were just *drinking buddies* that gravitated away. The ending of those particular friendships has been beneficial. I no longer have to deal with their drunken dramas. No more calls asking me to go out and get wild (and ultimately waste money that I can ill afford). No more listening to bullshit about fights, family issues and excuses. No more calls for a ride; not for a safe ride home from the bar, but to get places because they don't have gas money or can no longer drive (DUI). No more deadbeat *friends* asking for money or for loans (that they'll never pay back). Those are friends that I can honestly say I don't miss.

I've also had to release some very good friends from my life, or I should say that I've had to make myself unavailable to some very good friends, which does sadden me. There are a few people who I deeply love and care intensely about, but being around them isn't good for my sobriety. They don't tempt me or have a bad influence on me, but drinking is such a major part of their lives that I feel uncomfortable being around them. I see what they are doing to themselves, to their own financial situation and the impressions they are leaving on their children. I care for them so much that when I'm with them I find myself tempted to help them see what they're doing to themselves. That is not my responsibility. Could I just hang out with them, enjoy their company and friendship? Probably. But when their entire entertainment, relaxation and social world is focused around drinking, I have nothing in common with them and it's no longer fun for me. So I had to make the decision not to continue the friendship. I don't miss the drama but I do miss certain aspects of the friendships; closeness, intimacy, a warm bond, conversation and human interaction. But I have an obligation to myself to maintain and preserve my sobriety.

I have become much closer with other friends. For instance, people whom I've known for many years, but was never really close with, have become dear friends. It turns out that they like me more as a sober person. They always liked me, but my heavy drinking made them feel uncomfortable. (Sounds similar to what I just mentioned in the preceding paragraph, doesn't it?) I was never aware of how they felt. I found out by having lucid conversations with them. These are people who I had always admired but didn't hang out a lot because they either weren't heavy drinkers c they didn't drink at all. My own drinking behavior limited the kinds of friends that I would associate with.

As a sober person, my choice of friends is far greater than when I was a drinker. Think about what I just said. When you're a drunk, you *think* you have a lot of friends, but it's actually limited to only other drunks. Those are conditional friends – based on the condition that you drink with them. Once you start living sober, your friend pool becomes unlimited. I never realized this, nor would I have believed it had I not experienced it for myself. You can still hang out with drunken friends, but why? As a sober person you can hang around more types of people: occasional drinkers, legitimate social drinkers and other non-drinkers.

The following segment may sound repetitive, but it covers a few different aspects of friendships when you sober up. It is excerpted from; *Living Sober Sucks.*

> Some of your *friends* may not want to hang out with you anymore, and you may find that you don't want to hang out with them anymore. They may act differently around you, feel nervous around you. Some will become fearful of you because they can sense the personal power you posses - which makes some people jealous and hateful towards you. Revel in knowing that you are powerful and can control yourself. Be ready for the brutal truth that some friendships and relationships may completely fall apart when you sober up, while other relationships will become deeper, stronger, healthier and more emotionally intimate. This is when you will find out who your friends really are, what they are made of, and how much you can count on them. You will also find out what kind of friend you are to other people. If your friends don't want to help you, it may be because this

#7) Parties, events and social gatherings

"Every party needs a pooper, that's why we invited you."
Anonymous

If you want to be a wet blanket at parties, events and social gatherings – go ahead. At least you won't have to worry about being tempted to drink in the future, because you won't be invited back. If you don't want to go places where alcohol is served, that's your choice. If you never want to go to a concert, festival, comedy club, bowling alley, wedding reception, whatever – that's your choice. But why would you want to rob yourself of all that fun?

I'll grant you that it's not a good idea to attend Oktoberfest on Day 2 of your sobriety, but eventually you'll want to, or have to, attend some function where alcohol is served. Unless of course you plan on hiding from the rest of the world and never going to a wedding reception, never going to a festival or fair, or never going to a restaurant that might serve – God forbid – wine! You'll also have to never watch a Football, Basketball or Baseball game on TV.

You have to prepare yourself for all of these tempting situations if you plan on living a normal, fully engaged life. Sure, you can go sit in the "alcohol free" section at Baseball and Football games, but you're going to have to walk through the parking lot and through the turnstiles, then past all the concession areas. Sooner or later you're going to have to pee. What are you going to do? Have someone put a pillowcase over your head and walk you to your

...r to the bathroom? (I went to the Symphony and there were ...e vendors in the lobby.) Virtually any public place or ...tertainment venue you go to will have alcohol for sale. You ...etter get used to it.

In this chapter I want to pass along some ideas on how to enjoy yourself when you inevitably encounter alcohol out in the real world. These are ideas to get you thinking. I'll try to cover most common areas that you might come across but you'll have to plan, act and react on your own.

Go with a sober friend: Ask a sober friend to go along with you to events. If you have a spouse or partner, talk about your need for their support – before the event. You're not making it their responsibility to keep you sober – you're letting them know that you want to enjoy the event with them and that you would really appreciate their help. If it's a good friend, spouse or partner, (and they happen to be social drinkers), it's not unreasonable for you to ask them to refrain from drinking or to limit it to a few. For whatever reason, maybe you don't have a spouse or sober friends to go with you. You can still go and use the opportunity to meet some new sober friends.

Make an agreement: If you do bring a sober friend, then make an agreement. The agreement could be, "We're going to have fun and not whine about not being able to drink." You could also make the agreement that they can tug your arm, nudge your foot or give you some signal when it's time to move away from a certain crowd or if one of you starts talking too self-righteous with a group. You can also make an agreement with yourself such as, "I won't be a downer. I'm going to have fun. I won't feel sorry for myself. If I get tempted I'll leave early. For every drink I turn down, I'll make sure that I reward myself (friend/spouse) with something special."

Watch the show: Don't just watch the show or event you're attending, but watch the show that's taking place *all around you.* As I mentioned in Chapter #1, you don't want to be fixated on watching how much everyone is drinking. In this instance I'm talking about watching the dynamics that take place and (sometimes) the wreckage that ensues. I love going to wedding receptions and placing bets, not for money but for fun, on who will fall over first. I like to watch as the "loving couple" across from me turns into a raging brawl after two hours of drinking. At one wedding in particular, I had a drunk guy say to me, "Dude, I own the dance floor. Every one of these bitches wants to fuck me." Within twenty minutes of saying that he was falling over, could barely walk and was being forcibly escorted out the door (bitch-less).

I find watching all that is going on around me is a fascinating study in human behavior. I watch as the body language changes and becomes more animated, as the co-ordination slowly ebbs away. Watching as some dopey guy, who now thinks he looks like Adonis, is pawing and crawling on a woman that would never be caught dead with him – but he can't figure it out – and then calls her "bitch" for rebuffing him. There is so much to watch if you just look a bit closer.

Watching other people helps reinforce my desire to stay sober. I begin to wonder if that's how I behaved? It reaffirms that I never want to be like that ever again. By watching those around me I am able to prepare myself better if I am approached by a drunken person or if I am going to engage with a drunk. If they're drunk, I can preplan my escape, have my "no thanks" statements ready and limit how much conversation I want to participate in. I'm not prejudging people or being prejudiced, but by watching people closer I'm more tuned into their behaviors and can interact with them better.

As you're watching the show around you, you might notice some other people who aren't drinking. Gravitate towards them and introduce yourself. It's not as scary as you think to introduce yourself to someone. You could walk up to them and say, "Seems a bit safer over here, everybody's pretty drunk over there." Then listen to how they react. You might make some new friends or you might find them to be boring. You won't know until you know.

Do some mental math: I'm also fascinated by how much money is exchanged during the act of drinking. I like watching people argue over the bar bill. "I only had two beers, you drank shots, so you have to pay more." It's funny to see the stunned faces on people when their bar tab arrives. Watch as the cheap guy has to keep digging in his wallet when he's plying a woman with drinks. See people who can ill afford to buy one beer buying a round for their friends.

I make a game out of it. In my head, I try to figure out how much money is being exchanged. For instance; how much do I think that table's bar bill will be? How much has that guy spent on drinks trying to get that woman's phone number? When the beer vendor passes four bottles down the row; how much did the person spend including tip? How much have I not spent? Maybe I'll go get a team jersey or some other treat with the money I didn't spend on beer. My goal isn't to be cheap but to fully enjoy what limited financial resources I have. I want to reward myself for not drinking and for not spending more than I can afford.

Keep your mouth shut and act normal: Don't preach or lecture others that do drink. Mind your own business. Don't feel obligated to spread the good word of sobriety. I'll be going into greater detail about this in Chapter #12, but right now I'll briefly touch on ways to conduct yourself at public events.

The more naturally you behave, the more comfortable people will feel around you and they in turn will behave more naturally. You don't have to go into graphic detail about your drinking past and wreckage when talking with people. You can simply tell them, "I don't drink anymore." If they ask why, use your own judgment. Talk with them about it if they seem genuinely curious, but you can also say, "It just wasn't good for me. We can talk about it some other time. What's exciting in your life?" Find out about them, talk about anything else other than your drinking past. This isn't hiding from issues or lying, it's just being normal. Who wants to hear about your ugly past at a party? If you disclose a lot of sordid details you're just giving them gossip material. That's not a criticism of humanity; people are social beings and we like to gossip (or at least discuss our observations of others if you don't want to call it gossiping).

Speaking of gossiping, you can always talk about your observation of others to the person you're with. As I mentioned earlier, I like to watch the show. I joke with the people I'm with about, "Look at how hammered that woman is getting," or "Can that guy act any sleazier?" It's not all criticizing gossip, I notice and point out other people who appear to be having a good time. We might even joke about our own past behaviors, tell stories about dumb shit we've done, but I try to not come off as self-righteous.

Parties, events and social gatherings (especially if you are a guest) are not to be used as a platform to educate others about sobriety and it's not your place to do so. It's tempting to get involved when you see someone getting too drunk. Depending on the circumstances, you could privately tell the host, "I think Jim is pretty drunk. Does he have a ride? I'd hate to see him hurt someone or get arrested," then leave it at that. You don't have to become the self-appointed savior.

If you're at a public venue such as a concert, festival, show, whatever, and someone is getting drunk and disturbing you or disrupting your enjoyment of the event, then go talk to security about it. Don't take it upon yourself to control or correct the other person. This can jeopardize your safety if you try to confront a drunk. Let security or the staff take care of it. Additionally, don't take it upon yourself to go on a witch hunt – looking for drunks to have them kicked out. A drunk (presumably) paid the same as you did to get in. Let them enjoy the event how they want to.

When it comes to parties, events and social gatherings, if the environment bothers you, if someone makes you feel uncomfortable – then get away from them or leave. This may not seem fair, but would you rather be safe and sober or risk relapse? The choice is yours.

Alcohol alternatives: If you've ever gone to a restaurant (that serves alcohol) the first thing your waiter or waitress will ask is, "Can I get you a cocktail or something to drink?" If it's a Sports Bar or someplace that's known for their unique beers, they'll go over a list of all their special craft brews. A Mexican restaurant will push their Margaritas or some other concoction. At finer restaurants you'll probably be handed a wine list with the menu. So what? That's how they make money and it's a legal product. You don't have to make a scene, you don't have to say anything other than, "Well those sound good but I'll have a coffee (Coke, Iced Tea, whatever)." "Water's fine," works pretty good too. You don't have to make an announcement that you don't drink. Just because you're not drinking shouldn't change the quality of service. In fact, you can get the special dish that you really want, some appetizers or you can tip a bit extra for good service with the money you're saving.

For the most part, people are just being gracious when they offer you a drink. Someone who has never met you has no idea what your history with alcohol is. Offering you a drink or a beer is socially acceptable. Even people who know that I don't drink will unconsciously say, "Hey can I get you a beer or something?" I don't get shitty with them, I simply say, "No thanks." If I'm at a picnic or go to a neighbor's house, I'll typically carry a bottle of water (in a can-koozie). That way I'm already set in the event I'm offered a drink.

There are certain social events (weddings, dinner parties, etc.) where you might want to have what *appears* to be a drink in your hand. This could be a way of helping you feel more normal and it will keep an overly gracious host and other guests from asking if you need anything. Like I just mentioned, people aren't purposefully trying to get you to crack, offering someone a drink is socially acceptable and it's an easy way to start a conversation with someone (you) that they don't know. Additionally, most people won't care whether you're drinking alcohol or not, they're just looking to see if they can get you something.

Some people like to openly carry a bottle of water as a way of making a statement. Do whatever you want. I prefer to just look like an average person at a party. I like to order my own "drink" from the bar. That way I can ask the bartender directly for what I want and I don't have to concern myself with explaining to anyone why I want a seltzer (that is if they were to even ask). When I order my non-alcoholic drink I specifically request that it be in a regular drink glass, not a big cup with a straw. If I'm at a picnic, festival or event where beer is served in bottles/cans, I may buy a bottle and pour the beer out and re-fill it with water (providing that it's not a clear bottle).

Here are a few examples of drinks that look like alcohol:

- Seltzer or Tonic water with a twist of lemon
- Coke with a twist of lime
- Orange juice on the rocks
- Cranberry juice on the rocks
- A glass or mug of NA beer
- A bottle of NA beer (most people won't look at the label)

If I'm asked to join in with a round of shots, I just offer mine to someone else instead of turning the person down. I might say some ridiculously wild thing, "Aw thanks but Jaeger gives me the shits," or "No, I got really sick off that stuff once. I can't touch it." I know a guy who talks to the bartender beforehand. The bartender will give HIM a shot of Coke when he pours everyone else their shot. Answer however you want, but remember that the person who is extending the offer of a shot or a drink is doing just that; offering you a gift, they're not purposefully trying to get you to relapse.

Much of this might sound as if I'm being overly self-conscious, because as I said, most other people don't care whether you're drinking or not. I do all of this for me; so that *I feel* as if I fit in. It truly does keep a lot of gracious offers and nosy people at bay, especially the other drunks. Other drunks want you to drink with them. If other drunks keep pushing and prodding me, I have no problem walking away from them. If it's a situation where they're part of the group or for whatever reason I can't walk away from them, I have no problem being impolite and politically incorrect. I will come right out and say, "Leave me alone," or something even more direct like, "Fuck off," if the conditions warrant it. I have to preserve and protect my own sobriety.

Summary: All these ideas sound great: bring a sober friend, watch the show, keep your mouth shut, act normal, etc. Real life doesn't always cooperate with your plans. People get drunk, shit gets crazy, the unexpected happens. It is ultimately your own responsibility to be responsible for your own behaviors and how you act. You can go out in life and have fun or you can mope. If you mope, you're only robbing yourself and robbing others of getting to know the fun, sober you. There will be struggles and temptations. It will be difficult and unsettling at times. You never know what public event or social gathering you'll be at when someone offers you a drink or other drunks want you to drink with them. Prepare yourself for the inevitable. You may have to leave parties, events and social gatherings early or pass on some tempting invitations. It sucks, but this isn't a game – this is preservation of your life.

Social gathering Worksheet:

Do I truly enjoy myself at social gatherings?: _____

What strategies can I use to enjoy myself better?: _____

_____

_____

Do I mind my own business and just enjoy the "show"?: _____

Have I learned techniques so I blend in naturally with the crowd?: ____

_____

_____

Do I have pre-planned responses to drink offers?: _____

What are those responses?: _____

_____

_____

_____

Do I spend time thinking of my sobriety *before* I go into an event?: ____

What are some statements or reminders I can think on *before* events?:

_____

_____

_____

_____

#8) Finding new sober friends

"I would rather be respected than be liked." – Mark A. Tuschel

It isn't necessarily *where* you go to meet new sober friends, it's more important *how you behave* and *how you present yourself*. Before I begin giving ideas for places you can go to meet new sober friends, I first want to talk about your own body language and being approachable. These are habits you can incorporate into your daily behavior that will benefit you in many ways, regardless of whether you're trying to meet new friends, dealing with old friends, or just standing in line at the grocery store.

Smile and laugh: Plenty of studies and research have been done on the psychological and physiological benefits of smiling and laughter. For the purposes of this chapter I'm going to talk about those benefits and not cite all the individual studies. If you're so inclined, you can look them up and research them yourself, (it'll give you something to do when you're bored).

Smiling is contagious, regardless whether it's a fake or genuine smile. When you smile, others will smile back at you. The best smiles are genuine and involve all of your face muscles and not just the muscles around your mouth. When you smile you don't appear as dower and others will be more willing to talk with you. It doesn't matter if you're driving your car, waiting in line, walking into a program meeting, wherever – smile. You'll truly feel better about yourself and others will spend more time looking at you. Research into smiling has shown that most people will avoid other people who don't smile. If you don't smile, people won't be as likely to make eye contact with you, they will gaze the other direction and purposefully walk around you. Smiling with another person creates a bond, because smiling is a non-combative, almost submissive gesture. When you smile you're letting the other person know that you are not a threat.

Smiling is good for your physical health and your psychological health. It makes you look more approachable and you will feel comfortable when approaching others. I consistently practice having a genuine smile, appearing happy and giving off body language signals that show that I am at ease. I am pleasantly surprised by how many people initiate conversations, approach me or are willing to engage with me when I inquire about them. If you're unsure of your smile, then practice in a mirror to get an idea of how you physically appear when you smile.

Smiling and laughing release endorphins into your bloodstream (laughter much more so than just smiling). Remember when I mentioned endorphins in Chapter #5? Endorphins are very similar in chemical make-up and effect as heroin or morphine, which relax the mind and body. This is why laughing hard gives you a natural high. People who aren't able to laugh naturally at things will often turn to drinking to release their inhibitions to enable themselves to smile and laugh, hence getting an endorphin rush. If smiling and laughing don't come naturally to you, prolonged use of alcohol won't make you a happy person. It can actually make unhappy people become more depressed.

If you are the type of person who used alcohol as a social crutch to help you smile and laugh, then eliminating alcohol consumption will make you *think* you're sadder than when you drank and you'll laugh less. So how do you overcome this? As hokey as it sounds, you have to force yourself to smile. Doing this honestly does have a positive effect on your autonomic nervous system and small amounts of endorphins will be released by your brain. Smiling makes it easier to laugh. And laughing is easier to do when you're around other smiling and laughing people. Plain and simple, if you're surrounded by grumpy, miserable, unsmiling people, how do you think you're going to feel? Your smile can make others smile, your laughter will help others laugh, and this creates a bond between the two of you and then you'll both feel better. Just the simple act of smiling is a powerful way to meet new friends.

Where to go: A lot of newbies are under the impression that the only place to meet new sober friends is at AA meetings. Going to meetings doesn't guarantee that the people you meet will be sober. Consider some of these details: Many people attending meetings are there because they are *trying* to quit drinking. This means that they are in the same weakened state that you are and it's easier than you think to talk each other into relapse. Some newbies aren't very experienced at living sober and probably won't have any tangible real life sobriety strategies to share with you. Other attendees may be court ordered or forced to be there; they aren't looking for fellowship, they're just serving time. Others simply want you to keep returning to meetings and not expand your circle of friends (there can be numerous reasons for this). Some people are there strictly to prey on the weak and vulnerable. I have witnessed it and I've even had people privately tell me, "Dude, I get laid all the time coming to these meetings." This is the unspoken, "13th Step."

I bring this up not to talk you out of attending AA meetings, but to pass along a word of caution. Go to meetings if you get something out of them, but don't go there with the explicit intent of meeting new friends. Then all you're doing (as some others do), is using meetings as a sober pick-up joint. So if you go to meetings, try to engage in the conversations. Go to different meeting locations. Be willing to help clean up after meetings. Be open to go with a group of people for coffee after a meeting. Who knows, you might find the perfect group that you're comfortable with. You won't know until you try. And remember to smile.

Other than AA meetings, there are plenty of places to go where you can meet sober people. I would like to refer back to Chapter #5. You can meet a lot of new sober friends by joining and being active at a health club or gym. Team sports and league sports (formed at or through the gym) are another possibility. I mention joining leagues through a gym because a lot of sports teams are sponsored by bars. This doesn't mean you shouldn't join them, but at least be aware that many of the games will take place at sports bars and team parties will be held at sponsoring bars.

Most hobbies have gatherings or hold conventions. Spend some time doing internet searches for your sport or hobby of interest. You might even google search the phrase "Sober Baseball Leagues" or whatever your favorite sport is. In Chapter #4 I talked about furthering your mind. You can go sit at a library or a Barnes & Noble and read books. You can go to a Starbucks, get a cup of coffee and sit there and read. If you're hoping to meet new friends at these places you will have to talk with people, introduce yourself, ask genuine questions about them and remember to smile.

Just because you don't drink doesn't mean you can't go out in public or go out and have fun. Fairs, festivals, concerts, sporting events all draw a wide variety of people. Pay attention to the people around you. Are they behaving like they're drunk? Do they have a beer in their hands? Watch for body language and indicators that someone else isn't drinking, then engage in some simple conversation. If you like to dance, you can still go out dancing or clubbing and not drink. If you're single you can still go wild and take home randoms, but you might find that the randoms you take home aren't very entertaining. Just by living sober you'll probably start making better choices about the type of people you befriend.

New sober friends aren't going to come running your way. You absolutely will have to try new things and you will risk failure, disappointment and rejection. You have to be open to meeting new people and everyone you meet doesn't have to become your new best friend. Really good, solid, healthy friendships take time to develop. And before you can find and attract good friends you have to learn to be a good friend yourself. The best person to practice good friendship with is yourself. If you love and respect yourself, this will carry over into how you treat other people. Of course it's a wonderful feeling to be in demand, to be desired, to be sought after, appreciated and respected - but only if it's because you're a good person and a good friend and not because you always pay the bar bill or you have good drugs

People you already know: If you actually look closely around you, you will most likely see that you do have a lot of friends. I surprise myself when I actually stop and view what is going on in my life. I may *feel* alone, but then I can see that I have numerous friends who I can call, email or go hang out with. I must make it a point to invite them into my life or ask to join theirs.

Look around you and pay attention to the people in your immediate world. There may be a lot of people you work with that don't drink, but you never noticed them before because they didn't go hang out at the bar after work, or you thought they were dorks because they never sat around at lunch kvetching and gossiping with the drinking crowd. I'm serious about this. If you just pay attention to the people you already know, watch how they behave and listen to the types of things that they talk about, you'll probably find a lot of new sober friends. But you will have to be the one to take the initiative, smile and talk with them.

Another part of hanging out with and befriending people you already know is that you must accept that other people *will* and *can* drink. It would be nice if there was an "acceptance pill"; something

103

you could take so it wouldn't bother you when other people drink, but there isn't, so you have to make the mental choice of acceptance yourself. You have to consciously tolerate them, and if they bother you or if it's too much of a struggle to be around people that drink socially, then you have to look for other friends. You ultimately have to preserve and protect yourself.

When it comes to friends, regardless of whether they're sober or drinkers, if neither of us gains something through knowing each other, then it is just a useless acquaintanceship and a waste of our time. I would rather spend my time alone than waste my life with someone just for the sake of being with someone. My time is too valuable to squander it on useless acquaintances.

Go public: You might think, "I can't do that, I don't want to be embarrassed." You don't think being drunk wasn't embarrassing? Chances are pretty good that anyone you were close with was already well aware of your condition. Some of these people may have drifted away or abandoned you because of your drinking. You might want to call or email some of your old, long lost acquaintances and tell them that you no longer drink. You may have told them this a million times in the past, so don't expect everyone to be all excited or even believe you. Your actions and behaviors are what will tell the truth. At least extending the offer to get together might help rekindle your friendship with them and you won't have to go searching all over for new friends.

Another way of you going public with your sobriety is being involved in social medias. Take facebook for example. If you go public and say that you're living sober and want to hang out with other sober people, you might be pleasantly surprised at how many of your facebook friends congratulate you and now suddenly invite you to events. I'm not guaranteeing that this will happen, but you don't know if you don't try. There are many websites which offer forums for writing about sobriety. You can also start your own blog and write about sobriety. You might gain a big following and meet people through your writing.

Spend some alone time: It may be a painfully lonely time for you, but then again it might not. It isn't necessarily that you are alone, but sobriety is unlike any way of life that you may be accustomed to – it's different – so it may *feel* like you're alone. It's natural to think, "Oh why did I do this? I had so many friends when I was drinking and now I'm lonely and I don't have any friends." But what were those friendships based on? Many were simply acquaintances that revolved around drinking. That doesn't mean that everybody who drinks is a bad friend, but you have to pay close attention to what's in your own self interest.

Time spent with one's self may feel lonely and unrewarding, but you are going through a discovery process. When you discover yourself and learn to value yourself, you won't feel the need to give your friendship away to just anybody. I'll admit that being alone allows the mind to wander and we begin to feel self-pity. That's when you'll turn to your *Secret Support Group*, detailed in the next chapter.

No one else but YOU can keep you sober, which is strange, because other people can pressure you into drinking. I'm not blaming those other people, you still have the power to choose, but your friends, peers, family and partners play a big role in influencing your own choices. Again, I'm not saying that all your friends that drink are bad friends. Each relationship is unique for you in its own special way. I have friends who I used to drink heavily with – we're still friends, they're still good people, and if I want to hang out with them then I must accept that they are going to drink. But if they're a negative influence and they don't respect my sober lifestyle, then I must make the choice to stay away from them.

I'm sorry, but there will be some lonely times. The reality is that you will drift away from some friends, and other friends will gravitate towards you and your new lifestyle. And as I said, I would rather spend time alone, with myself, than to compromise my health, my mind, my finances and my ethics, just to be accepted and called "friend" by a bunch of drunken fucks. I know I sound crude, but I value and respect myself too much, and I would like you to value and respect yourself as well. You are the only one that has to live your life; no one else will do it for you.

Summary: There is going to be a period of transition, leaving some old friends and acquiring new ones. This does not mean that you resign yourself to a life of loneliness; hiding from the world. Most people are social beings and we want to be around others. Searching for replacement friends can be just as dangerous and destructive as searching for a replacement to getting drunk. Your friends and peers play a larger role in influencing your sobriety than you realize or care to admit. Respect yourself and value yourself, don't give your friendship away to just anyone. Every person you meet does not have to become you new best friend. Take the time to get to know people and let them get to know you.

A major aspect to having good friendships is that you also have to be a good friend in return. Ask yourself objective questions: Would I want to hang out with me? Am I fun to be around or am I always whining and complaining? Do I leach off of my friends, emotionally or financially? Do I offer anything in return within the friendship? Do I *expect* people to be my friend? Do I put *conditions* on my friendships?

Pay close attention to your body language and your smiling. If you look grumpy, you'll feel grumpy. You want to appear approachable. When you look approachable, others will be willing to get to know you. Don't just wait for people to come and talk to you, take the initiative to talk with them. It would be nice if people came running your way, just wanting to be your friend. That can happen, but only once people know who you are. If you want new sober friends, be a good sober friend yourself. You have to smile, be willing to laugh, take some risks, extend your friendship and go discover who's out there in this world.

Friend finder Worksheet:

Who are some people I already know that I would like to be closer friends with?: _____

_____

Why would I like to be closer with them?: _____

_____

Who do I work with that I would like to get to know better?: _____

_____

_____

Why do I want to get to know them better?: _____

_____

What can I do to make myself a better friend?: _____

_____

_____

What can I do to make myself appear friendlier and approachable?: ____

_____

_____

Do I present myself as friendly?: _____

Do I smile and laugh?: _____

Am I willing to introduce myself to people?: _____

Where can I go, or what can I do to meet new sober friends?: _____

_____

_____

#9) Do you need AA or God?

"The day I needed God and looked for Her, She called in sick."
Mark A. Tuschel

One size does not fit all, regardless of whether it's shoes, a swimsuit or a recovery system. Here's an example. The United States Foreign Policy is to try and make all other countries a democracy just like ours. The same free market system, same judicial system, same multiparty political system, etc. That's a great idea, but it doesn't always work. Every country is different with different cultures, history and social norms. It took the United States over 200 years to get to where we are now. It often fails when we try to make other countries be "just like us" in 30 days. We can lead and show by example, but we can't force the changes we desire.

Forcing a belief system on someone can make them cooperate for a while, but eventually they want to do their own thing. They might rebel, revolt and revert back to what they were or worse than they were in the first place. When the United States assists but allows another country to customize their own plan, that country often finds a unique system that is successful for them.

Re-Invention is similar. A regimented system may work perfectly for some. A modified version of a regimented system may work better for others. And a customized plan, using parts of many systems, may work best for other people. Problems arise when those who believe in a certain system don't welcome or

111

support others who don't believe or follow their system to the letter. Both parties want the same thing; to stay sober and support each other, but a closed-minded belief results in a "you will fail if you don't follow my system" attitude.

As an individual you can accept and welcome others into your circle, even if the other person doesn't believe the exact same things you do. That doesn't infer that you (the believer) have to change or compromise your own beliefs, you just accept that another person has a different viewpoint. You then show by example and maintain comfort in your own beliefs.

The danger of joining or buying into a certain belief system is that other members can fill your head with false expectations. They may not be purposefully lying, but they want you to believe in the same things as they do. They want you to believe that everything will automatically work out for the best, but only if you follow their belief system. For instance: "Follow the steps and the steps will work." "Let go and let God." "Your Higher Power (God, Buddha, Jehovah, Yahweh, Allah, whoever) will give you answers and guide you."

What you're doing is relinquishing your power and decision making authority over to some invisible, bearded, make-believe friend in the sky. Then when difficulties or catastrophe strikes you feel abandoned. "Why did God do this to me?" Or you get yourself into the mistaken belief that "Everything will work out for the best." Then when it doesn't or you are struggling with temptation or relapse you think, "I thought this was supposed to work? How come it isn't? Everyone told me it would. What's wrong with me? I must be weak and flawed." Disenchantment or bitterness sets in. You lose self-confidence and self-esteem. You begin to question yourself, the program and the steps. Then you are told, "You didn't follow the steps. If you work the steps the steps will work."

Someone else's system, plan and beliefs may not work for you. You should even question the words I write in this book, then decide for yourself what you want to try, what might work best for you. No one else can live your life for you but you.

This takes me to my beliefs regarding God. I don't believe in a religious deity. (Go ahead, curse me now and pray that I will be smited.) Just because I don't believe in God, I would never judge you or tell you that you're wrong, weak, foolish or attempt to get you to reject your religious belief. When you believe in or follow a religion by your own choosing I respect that, and I would hope that you respect my position. I am not going to insult religion or ask you to question your faith. What I am going to do is ask you to be more personally responsible for your own life and pass a few words of caution along. These are my opinions and I welcome you to disagree with me.

Do not *expect* God to fix you or your problems. You can turn to your faith and religious doctrine for guidance, comfort and insight, but do not expect someone else to do the work for you. Relying solely on the belief that God will handle everything places you in a weakened position. You may not be as willing to fight for your own self preservation. For instance, when something bad happens and the person responds with, "Well, it was God's will," they are openly admitting that they have no personal control over conditions in their own life. They forego the process of rational analyzation. They don't think, "What were the events or conditions that caused this to happen? How can I fix it? What can I do to make the best out of this? What did I possibly do wrong?" along with numerous other questions that could be asked to get a better understanding and have some control of future outcomes.

When people say, "It was God's will," it implies that God is either punishing or rewarding you personally for some behavior or action that you have performed and God is doing this without telling you why. This attitude causes someone to believe that they are not completely responsible for various outcomes or occurrences. They neglect to take variables and randomness into account. It is grandiose thinking to believe that God would alter the universe and other people's lives to either reward or punish one individual. When something good that a person hopes for doesn't happen, they have unfounded feelings of guilt and unworthiness, "God didn't want this for me." This is highly detrimental to a person's self-esteem and they neglect to consider factual causes.

Most religions state that, "God has given you a free will," but then profess in their teachings that God has a plan for you and that God wants you to behave certain ways and perform certain activities to carry out His will. I happen to think that an individual can be a member of an organized religion, believe in God and still take full responsibility for their own lives. They can hold themselves in high self-esteem and be proud of themselves while loving and honoring their God. Here is the best example that I can give: Instead of saying, "By the grace of God I am sober today," why not say, "For the grace of my God I live sober today." You are then behaving and acting out of reverence and love for your God as opposed to fearing God or not exhibiting pride and taking credit for your own behavior.

If you are religious or are a member of a church, do you attend services out of a sense of obligation or because you like it? Do you enjoy the service? Are you inspired by it, refreshed and feel peace for attending? Or do you hurry to get there, show up at the last minute, tap your foot incessantly until the end and then rush out after the service like you're a lead-blocker for the Green Bay Packers? You should attend services because they enrich you, because you love your God. Look, you ain't fooling your God if you show up and *act* like you're enjoying the service.

Now that I've alienated myself from AA and religious believers, I want to point out that I support AA and religion. I agree with the goal behind them; to assist others in finding support and comfort. I don't support forcing, cajoling, insulting intelligence or threatening. AA was created as a fellowship to help others with alcohol problems. It is an open organization. But even *they* have requirements for attending: You must admit that you are an alcoholic, that you are powerless, that there is a greater power than yourself and that you seek help. In essence it is an exclusive club, but it's supposed to be open to anyone and everyone.

Private groups, religions and associations are different. They have their own established rules and criteria for membership. If you join, you are agreeing to follow their rules. You can join, question their rules or beliefs within your own mind, but it is not appropriate for you to disrupt and unsettle other members who are there celebrating their faith or belief. You have the right to choose to no longer attend.

I have always stated that if you are serious about living sober you should spend the time investigating various systems, groups and programs. You will gain an education and you may discover a group or system that works for you. If you decide to attend religious services or AA meetings, then do so because you want to – not because someone else told you that you should or that their system is the only way.

Once again I would like to plagiarize from my other book; *Living Sober Sucks*. Here is an excerpt from Chapter #10:

> **Turning to God:** My goal in this section is not to persuade for or against any religious belief system, nor to debate the existence of a God or Deity. But I can't caution enough that during the initial sobering up time (30-90 days) you will be vulnerable to being influenced into spiritual beliefs.

115

Many people will tell you, "All you need to do is turn to God" or "Let go and let God" or "You HAVE to accept a higher power." Look, if you're not a believer in God - then don't suddenly start now - hoping that God will cure you. If you do that, you are just setting yourself up for a big letdown. God isn't going to cure you, I can't cure you - only YOU can cure you.

Many people believe that God will give them signs along the way. If this is your belief system - great - watch very closely for those signs from God. But God is only going to do so much - most of this will be up to you. If you have a strong religious foundation then use it to your own empowerment with sobriety. If you are a believer, you probably already know how to turn to God. Your God and your religion's teachings will give you something to turn to in times of trouble and temptation. You may want to consider delving deeper into your faith and becoming more active with its mission. If you have fallen away from your faith, this can be a perfect time to revisit it and get to know your God again. Most religious groups offer "Alcohol Free" get-togethers and support groups. Become a participant and actively celebrate your faith.

You cannot always burden your friends with your need to talk. There may be times when it's too late at night, or simply no one is available. You will need to start relying on your own strength. That's when you might want to try turning to God or learning about spirituality. But again I want to issue a warning of caution about becoming too religiously overzealous. It's easy to use religion as a substitute addiction and become obsessed with it. You don't want to be the person that everyone hides from because all you talk about is how God helped with your recovery. I would never chide anyone about their religious beliefs nor would I ever try to talk anyone OUT of their faith. But if you don't have a legitimately strong faith, you can't suddenly turn religious and expect God to keep you sober. A Minister once told me, "It's pretty easy to find Jesus in prison, but when you get out He's nowhere to be found." I believe the same can happen with recovering addicts. We find God for a short time when we first sober up, then forget all about Him if we relapse or go back to our old habits. If you are so moved, slowly learn how to pray and get to know a God. After six months, then join a church, synagogue, mosque or whatever your religion of choice is. Choose a religion when you are ready and then stick with it. Never expect or think that it's up to God, your spouse, partner, friend, family or boss to sober you up. You are in charge of yourself and sobriety is completely up to you.

"God doesn't want me to live this way." Here is my own belief: God does not meddle in the personal affairs and doings of his followers *or* dissenters. A fair and loving God does not show favoritism. God makes sure that the universe and nature keeps functioning. This is evidenced to me by the fact that even people who don't believe in God or follow a certain religion can still live fulfilling, moral lives. A God should be turned to for spiritual, emotional, social and moral guidance. I do not expect God to do my work for me or give me anything that She would not give to anyone else.

Develop your own secret support group. When I say, "secret support group" I'm not referring to an exclusive private club. I'm talking about having a group of friends that you can call or turn to when rough patches come along. The "secret" part is that they are unaware that they're in fact members and they're helping you. This isn't underhanded or manipulative. You will actually be expressing more interest in *them* than in your own problems.

People become tired of hearing you whine about the same problem over and over again. (This is the main reason that I never liked attending meetings; listening to the same person whine about the same problem week after week. Never growing, expanding or developing beyond the same issue every week.) If you keep complaining and whining about your alcohol issues and your problems with temptation, eventually people will get sick of listening to you. Their phone rings, they check the screen, "Oh, it's *him* again. I don't want to hear his shit anymore." You'll end up talking to more voicemail than live people. Do yourself and your friends a favor and quit bitching already.

To properly utilize your secret support group, you call your friend and ask how their life is or talk about anything other than your issues with alcohol. Expressing genuine interest in someone else will get your mind off your own problems. This isn't hiding from reality – this is called normal conversation. For instance, if I'm feeling down or feeling self-pity because I want to drink, I'll call a friend and the conversation will start off something like this:

"Hey Carl, it's Mark. So what's going on in your life? How've you been lately?" As the conversation progresses I'll ask him if he's seen any movies lately, any sporting events, gone on a vacation somewhere or ask for his impression of a recent news item. I will touch on my issues, but only if he asks. And I'll be cognizant of my demeanor. I won't suddenly get all melancholy, but I'll be honest. "Well, it's been a little rough lately, but that's why I call a friend like you. You have a way of distracting me and helping me feel better." I'm not avoiding reality or my problems, I'm just trying to live a normal life and talk with a friend about normal shit.

Summary: The theme of this chapter is to get you to think on your own, to make some decisions on your own. Many people will disagree with me and say, "Look where thinking on your own got you. You're a despicable drunk." Sure, your thinking may have been flawed in the past, but now that you're sober you do need to start thinking on your own behalf. You need to think in terms of self preservation. That may include going to meetings or joining a religious organization. But do that only because you want to, not because someone else said that you should. Don't expect God, AA or anyone else to cure you – only *you* can cure you. You can lean on people, but you will have to walk this path in your own shoes.

As I mentioned in the opening chapter, you don't have to accept (or constantly remind yourself) that you are weak, powerless, a hopeless eternal alcoholic, riddled with flaws and defects. You can if you want to – but why would anyone want to speak about themselves in those terms, especially if you've already turned your life around for the better or are working on turning your life around?

Spirituality Worksheet:

Do I feel the need to attend religious services?: _____

When I do attend, do I feel rejuvenated?: _____

Do I attended services or meetings out of a sense of obligation or guilt?:

_____

Have I investigated any religious organizations to see if I like them?:

_____

Have I attended different AA locations?: _____

Can I take some of the teachings, modify them and make them work for

me?: _____

Have I developed my own *secret support group*?: _____

Who are the people in my *secret support group*?: _____

_____

_____

Do I thank those people?: _____

Do I listen to them?: _____

Am I a whiner and depressing?: _____

If I am, how can I stop being that way?: _____

_____

_____

#10) Being comfortable with yourself

"You can run all your life, but you can never hide from yourself."
Mark A. Tuschel

If there are things that you don't like about yourself, then you'll have to change them. Most things are within your control – I said most. Skin color, race, gender, height or sexual preference are things that you can't change. However many of your unique characteristics and attributes are within your control. Weight, physical fitness, behaviors, education and financial status are things that you have the power to make decisions about and you do have a certain amount of control over. An honest accounting and an acceptance of some basic truths will help you make the most out of who you really are. Trying to be something or someone that you are not can lead you into compromising your own health and safety in order to be accepted.

We're all born with certain innate talents, or a knack at certain things that are unique to each one of us. Gaining control over things that you struggle with will bring feelings of accomplishment and pride. Other skills or talents that come naturally may not feel as rewarding, but you can still exploit your own inborn abilities to allow you to do the other things that you want. For instance, you might be a gifted musician, but playing musical instruments may not be your passion. You could pursue work as a studio musician or a music instructor to *earn a living*, but spend your private time enjoying your photography hobby.

Some characteristics aren't socially accepted and aren't in your best interest. For instance, "I'm lazy, I don't like commitments, I don't like to be honest, I don't want to work. I want to drink, party and have sex with as many people as I can." These might be your true desires, but they probably won't benefit you in the long run. All behaviors, actions and inactions come with consequences. If you're willing to accept the consequences of antisocial or unhealthy behavior, that's your choice. If you don't like the way you are or the way your conditions are, then you must change, but change requires work on your own behalf. When change is forced upon you or it happens by default, it's often less internal work to adapt to the forced change than when you want to initiate the change yourself.

"I want answers, not suggestions." Sorry, it's unreasonable for me to dictate what you should do to be comfortable with yourself. A big part of enjoying life sober is the discovery process, discovering what gives you pleasure, what you like doing and being yourself. That's not the case for everyone. Some people aren't as adventurous and prefer to stick with the habits, hobbies or interests that they were taught to like or exposed to while they were growing up. Some have to be told what to do and how to behave. Regardless of whether you want to experiment and discover, or stay within the boundaries of what you know and what you're familiar with, you're still being yourself.

Accepting yourself: Warts and all, you are you. There are some factual limitations to all of us. Be it physical stature, mental comprehension, learning capacity or talents. Understanding and embracing personal limitations will help you get the most out of your sobriety. I'm not inferring that you don't dream, have aspirations or try the unknown, but I refer back to Chapter #2: accepting the reality of feasibilities and probabilities. Drunken delusions and sober delusions are equally limiting.

124

Delusions cross over the fine line of *having* hopes and dreams to actually *believing* that these hopes and dreams are destined to happen or that they will happen without any finite plans or effort on your own behalf. Being delusional can cause *immobility*, where you just sit back and wait for things to happen. Being delusional can also cause you to *blame others* or make excuses for your circumstances. Even in the event you do take action, delusional thinking may get you doing the *wrong things*, literally wasting your time, performing activities in an attempt to reach unrealistic or highly improbable goals. I'll go over each one of these: immobility, blame and doing the wrong things.

Immobility comes from a belief that, "everything will work out somehow," then you sit back and wait for everything to fall into place. If you wait for "everything to work out," you will be sadly disappointed when it doesn't. Making things happen requires some element of effort on your own behalf. Even the simplest things require you to be a participant (at some level) in their outcome. An example would be winning the lottery. You can't win if you don't go through the simple act of buying a lottery ticket. I'm not suggesting or condoning that you buy lottery tickets, I'm just using this as an example. So don't be immobile. Be a participant, do some simple things and some wonderful things may come of it.

Placing blame on others for your failures is a way of avoiding and not acknowledging one's own limitations. We had a tendency to blame others for our drinking. Now we might bring this *blaming others* mentality over into our sobriety. "I sobered up and they didn't do this or that didn't happen." You're forgetting that sobriety alone doesn't guarantee shit. Sobriety will allow for a clearer thought process, but every sober thought doesn't guarantee correct decisions. Clear thinking *will* aid in accepting your own realistic limitations. Once you stop blaming others for your conditions and difficulties you'll begin to understand your own limitations (physical, mental, financial, geographical, etc.). You can then exploit your strengths and abilities and then work at making the most out of what you do have and what you are capable of doing. When you stop blaming others, you'll focus more on being a participant in the direction of your own life and won't just wait for "everything to work out."

Doing the right things can be difficult when your thinking is delusional. When you're delusional about an outcome or a desire, you invest your time, energy and activities towards achieving an improbable result. Again, I'm not saying that you don't try new things or pursue lofty goals, but spending all your time and effort in hopes of becoming a professional NBA player, when you're only 5'2", is a waste of your energy. Your talents can be productively applied elsewhere. This is in no way suggesting that you give up all hopes and dreams and accept whatever comes your way. Recognition of specific limitations will allow you to adapt and work around those limitations. Acknowledging those limitations will help you get over unwarranted feelings of inadequacy and allow you be more comfortable with yourself.

Accepting others: Being yourself doesn't mean that you behave and act in ways which show no concern for others. You can be yourself, hold your own beliefs and have your own opinions without damaging or taking away from another person. You want to show respect for the other person, but that doesn't mean you have to agree with them. In the event that you don't like someone, agree with their beliefs or care for their lifestyle, then stay away from them. An honest appraisal and acceptance of others will help you decide whether this person is supportive or destructive in your sobriety.

This all sounds great in a perfect world, but what if this person happens to be a family member, a co-worker, a customer or someone that you have to engage with? I refer back to establishing boundaries for yourself. Only allow yourself to engage within the parameters of what is required to get matters handled. You can still defend your position without being confrontational, "Well that's how you see it but I don't see it that way." Every conflict and personality difference doesn't turn out textbook perfect. Do the best you can to control yourself, learn from the situation, learn about the other person and make the best out of the conditions that exist. Remember that the other person has the same right as you do to believe whatever they want. Accepting others as they are will better help you accept yourself as you are.

Self-interest: Most people give the words selfish and self interest negative descriptions. Selfish is bad if you gain by purposefully causing someone else's loss, if you take what is not yours, if you do whatever you want regardless of how it may affect others and if you are not willing to share yourself with others. It's important to put these words in the proper context. Selfishness and self interest is *self preservation,* and it does not mean that it can only occur through someone else's loss or by harming someone else.

Self preservation is doing what is right for you. You should be focused on keeping yourself healthy, educated and doing things that give you a feeling of pride. That pride might come from being a good spouse or partner, a good employee, a good parent or for staying sober. Having pride in yourself, your work and your behavior are what build self-esteem.

Self preservation also means that you are willing to say "NO." Not saying "no" in a sense of greed or that you are not willing to share or be of help to others, but saying "no" for your own health, benefit and protection. "No, I'm not gonna go hang out with you guys, I gotta get home and help my kids with homework. No, I'm not going out clubbing getting all crazy with you. No, I'm not buying this 12-pack, bottle of wine, bottle of Vodka, whatever... I'm putting this money in an envelope and I'm taking it to the bank tomorrow." Self preservation means that you are willing to forego immediate gratification and do what is in your own best interest. Is this exciting or as fun as getting drunk? No. But self gratification usually comes at someone else's expense, and ultimately at your own expense.

Self preservation requires you to think. You will have to think on your own behalf and think of what's best for you. If you blindly follow the interests and directions of someone else, then you are at their mercy. You do what they tell you to do, go where they tell you to go, behave how they tell you to behave. And you do this because you think, "I want people to like me, I want a lot of friends." But who are you harming if you allow others to influence you and do what they want you to do? You might think you're being unselfish, but you're only harming yourself.

It is human nature to seek pleasure; but when the pleasure is self destructive and is only an escape from reality or from your own mind, then there is no real pleasure. Then we feel guilt, regrets, have no pride or no self-esteem and hopelessness. The misconception is that pleasure comes from over-abundance or from something external. Seeing the look of joy or respect on your child's, spouse's or your parent's face – can be pleasurable. It may not be as exciting as getting drunk, but it can be more gratifying and more rewarding to your soul.

YOU are the most important person in your life, followed by those that you love, care about or are responsible for. If you don't care for yourself, you will not be able to care for them. Be a bit selfish, be self interested, pursue pleasure, but also pursue self preservation. You can hide from shit all your life, but the results and the consequences are still taking place in the background. Life doesn't wait for you to get your shit together; it keeps going on whether you're paying attention or not.

The stigma of being a "recovered al
people will have certain beliefs about
impression of you if or when they find out
They often unconsciously think to them.
recovered alcoholic. He's a weak person." Th
like to tell people (if the subject comes up),
Alcoholic." This statement opens the door to a
conversation. The discussion isn't spent describin
wreckage or the trail of self destruction; it takes the
a positive direction. You can talk about your posi
where you currently are and how you currently beha
the topic of this stigma in greater detail in Chapter #12.

Getting over your guilt: Guilt is as an invisible barricad
you and being comfortable with yourself. When you feel
and shame for your past it's extremely difficult to be com
with how you are now. This doesn't mean that you
culpability for past behaviors or ignore your current conseque
from past actions. Accept what you were, accept what you h
created, done or caused. To fully enjoy being yourself, you m
forgive yourself, pay restitution if required and emancipa
yourself. The following is excerpted from *Living Sober Sucks*.

> "I want to free myself of all the remorse, the regrets, the
> wreckage, the damage I've done. I want to eliminate the
> pain - I want to pay my penance and clear the slate." I
> understand that it is natural to want to rid oneself of painful
> emotions. To make restitution to those you have wronged
> and make everything better again. Sorry to tell you this, but
> sometimes you can't get rid of these things - and who (or
> what) do you want to give this wreckage to anyway? Some
> things in life can't be undone. That doesn't mean that you
> have to live the rest of your life with guilt and sadness.

ou can free yourself of these feelings by accepting the reality that you are personally responsible for past actions. But the good part is you do not have to be controlled by past actions or past experiences. You want to learn from them and learn to not repeat them. As you live sober, you don't have to react in the ways you once did to situations because you won't be hiding inside of a bottle. For example, you don't have to argue or get into fights with people, you don't have to get involved in dangerous, risky or unhealthy activities. You won't ignore bills, problems or conflicts. You will address your problems head-on and they won't get out of your control.

If you feel as if you need to pay some sort of penance, the best way will be to live a sober and fulfilling life. Live happy and healthy for your partner, your children, your friends and yourself. Your penance may also include that you pay off your debts, pay child support, serve jail time or community service. Extend the olive branch and ask the people that are important to you what penance they would like of you. What can you do for *them* to clear your relationship? You don't have to do this with everyone. I believe that some things are better left unaddressed. Some people aren't worth the time and effort to make amends with. Some situations may be too painful to revisit - why open up old wounds? Again I will clarify that you shouldn't live in denial or hide from your past - some things in life cannot be undone - but you do not have to live and act based on what you have done or what has happened in your past. These things are only past experiences - and that's all they are.

The best way to *not* be controlled by your past is to *not* constantly re-live it. Don't keep thinking about it and don't tell everyone you meet your history. Retelling your history

will only remind you of it and replaying bad scenes from your life will not allow you to love yourself, love others and constructively move forward with your life. It is true that some of your past actions can't be undone. There may be factual conditions that must be dealt with - unplanned children, car accidents, fights, wasted money, ruined relationships, broken marriages, criminal records.

Accepting responsibility and dealing with things that have happened can be your penance. Ridding yourself of guilt requires conscious, positive, forward thinking by you. You can't keep blaming your parents, society or the injustices of others for your present condition. Blaming someone else or yourself will not solve your present problem or improve your future. Past experiences explain how you got to where you are and why you feel like you do. Where you go and how you approach your future is your own choice. You can visualize and think of yourself as the helpless victim of past experiences or you can visualize and plan for your future.

Summary: The theme of this chapter is for you to accept others and to accept yourself. Accepting yourself is not saying, "Oh I'm an alcoholic and I can't help what I do." That is a lame statement to deny your own responsibility and to avoid accepting who you really are. Simply doing whatever you want in life without taking other people into consideration is *bad selfishness*. Good selfishness is *self preservation;* doing what is in your own healthiest best interest. Being comfortable with yourself as a sober person means that you graciously accept that there are limitations to each one of us. Trying to be something you are not is a major factor for drinking. Thinking that you are something you are not is a delusional result of drinking. You are you. Understand and accept your limitations, then work around those limitations and make efforts to improve yourself. Enjoy what you are and become comfortable with sobriety.

<u>Being yourself Worksheet:</u>

What positive characteristics do I have?: _____

_____

_____

What can I do to get the most out of them?: _____

_____

_____

How would these characteristics benefit me?: _____

_____

_____

What positive characteristics haven't I been using enough?: _____

_____

_____

What positive characteristics would I like to have?: _____

_____

_____

How can I bring those characteristics into my daily actions?: _____

_____

What characteristics would I like to stop exhibiting?:_____

_____

_____

How will I control useless and destructive characteristics?: _____

_____

#11) Can I ever go back?

"No matter which way you put your hand in a blender, it's going to hurt. So don't put your hand back in the blender."
Mark A. Tuschel

Oh what a tempting thought, "Can I ever go back?" Maybe you could, but probably not. And go back to what? For what purpose? If you've ever known the joys of getting drunk (don't deny that at some point you did enjoy it), thoughts of becoming a social drinker will always be dancing around in your mind. Do I sound like I'm talking in terms of absolutes? Absolutely. Of all the former drunks I've communicated with (thousands of them), I have yet to meet someone who has been able to quit drinking for a while and then become a social drinker. But allow me to clarify what I believe to be the difference is between a social drinker and someone who has a problem with alcohol misuse.

Social drinkers don't rely on alcohol as a crutch. Yes, a responsible social drinker may get drunk on occasion. They may even use a couple drinks to help them loosen up for social engagements, have a drink after dinner, have a few beers at a ballgame, whatever. But social drinkers can stop at one or two. They're also able to say "no" when drinking wouldn't be a good idea – such as when they have to drive, hold an important conversation or face up to a difficulty. Their life doesn't revolve around drinking. They can do without it if they have to.

On the other hand, an alcohol *misuser* can't stop after a couple. Whether they consciously know it or not, their goal is to get drunk. They rely on drinking as a crutch, whatever their own unique need

135

for this crutch might be – problem avoidance, alleviate stress, attempting to become uninhibited, pursuing pleasure, whatever. They are dependent upon catching a buzz to feel and act normal (or what they think is normal). For us drunks, we develop a physical and/or psychological dependency on booze.

Moderation or abstinence: I want you to think which is best for you, moderation or abstinence? This question may surprise you because you might be under the impression that this book is anti-alcohol. I'm not anti-alcohol; I'm anti-fuckin' up your life. Alcohol is a fun product, if used within moderation and used at the appropriate times. It's even fun to get drunk occasionally – why do you think so many people do it? But for those of us who misuse, overuse or become dependent on alcohol, then getting drunk is a problem.

So let me get back to the original question: Which is best for you – moderation or abstinence? If you can learn to control yourself and learn to enjoy alcohol in moderation, that's fantastic! But moderation is a difficult skill to learn and adhere to. If you're a hard core drunk like I was, moderation is impossible. So if you're a drunk and you're thinking of moderation, I'm telling you that I don't believe moderation is gonna work. You might think it can work, but this is where you need to do some personal reflection.

Think about why you're reading this book. Think back about your drinking history; whenever you started to drink were you ever able to stop? If you were never able to stop, or didn't like stopping, then moderation will not work for you. Here's why: What is alcohol? A mind altering substance that does exactly what it's supposed to do, it alters your mind and your mood. Once you put enough, or even just a little bit of it, into your system, you can't think straight and you lose control over it. I'm not saying that absolutely for certain moderation won't work for you. I know plenty of people who are capable of moderating their alcohol intake. However, they *are* legitimate social drinkers. But even some of those people end up getting drunk when they weren't planning on it.

I have yet to meet someone who's had problems with destructive alcohol overuse be able to drink in moderation. Every drunk that I have met and talked with that tried moderation, eventually fell back into their old habits; only faster and worse than when they originally stopped. For these people, it is a far more horrible torture that they suffer. They know how they felt when they were sober, they liked the personal progress they were making with their lives, and then they drank. And then they not only felt like shit physically, they mentally and emotionally felt even worse about themselves. They hate that they're weak, they hate what they did and they even say they hate themselves, and that saps them of all their self-esteem. Then the psychological mind-battle kicks in, "Oh I'm weak, I'll never quit, I'll never be any good, I hate being like this, why do I do this, I'm such a piece of shit." That on-again, off-again, on-again cycle is torture on your body and your mind. So total abstinence seems to be the best option for most of us.

If you can make moderation work, that's wonderful. If you're going to try moderation, remember, it's a difficult skill to learn and adhere to. It's difficult because you've got to consciously plan this out *before* you take that first drink. You can't just say, "I'm not gonna get fucked up tonight." You have to be able to tell yourself, in fixed terms, *before* you go out, "I'm only going to have 2 beers." If you don't give yourself a fixed number, before you know what's happening, you're gonna get all fucked up!

With that said, lemme discuss for a minute, how you moderate. As I just mentioned, you have to determine *beforehand* how much you're going to allow yourself to drink. That might mean you only take a limited amount of money with you if you're going out or you only buy so much beer, wine or whatever at the store. You can ask a friend to act as a *personal reminder*, but then you're placing the responsibility on someone else, and what happens when they start reminding you? You're out, you're having fun, everybody's having a great time, friends are buying you shots, and suddenly you're drunk before you know it. Then your *personal reminder* friend steps in and reminds you that you weren't going to get drunk. That can get ugly. The next thing you know, you're arguing with your friend. Or if you're drinking at home, all of a sudden you're heading out of the house at 11:30 at night to get more booze before the stores close, driving around when you're half in the bag. You think I'm making this shit up? No, I've done it. Once you start copping a buzz, the best laid plans get completely derailed.

And really, is moderation even any fun when it comes to certain things like drinking or drugs? Is it fun to do just a little "taste" of cocaine? Fuck no! At least not for me. I wanna do a mountain of the shit. Ask anybody who's trying to quit smoking or is dieting. Is it fun to have just two cigarettes a day, or to constantly keep tabs on every crumb they eat? No! They wanna smoke like Joe Camel and eat everything they can get their face near. Many people who moderate find that their every waking moment, their every thought is waiting for their time to get their junk. Watching the clock, waiting for 5pm to have that cigarette, then watching the clock and waiting for 10pm to have that next cigarette. That is pure self-imposed mental torture. So for many of us, the best answer, for our physical, social and mental health is abstinence.

Relapse: I've heard from plenty of people who have relapsed because they thought they could drink in moderation. They call me or email me cryin' the blues. I don't feel sorry for them, I feel *sad* for them, sad because I can tell how badly they wanted to keep this under control. But it didn't work. Some are hoping I'll say, "Aw that's okay, we all fuck up, you can try again." I might say *something* like that, but I'm not gonna be a "permission giver." Instead, I'm gonna say, "Yeah, we all fuck up, you can start over, but you can't keep tempting fate. You've proven to yourself that you can't control this shit once it's in your system. So the only way you can control alcohol is to abstain from alcohol. But that's only if you're serious about this." That might sound kind of mean, but if you keep getting coddled and told, "Oh it's okay, you'll figure it out," you will never change and you will always seek other permission givers. You'll make sure that you surround yourself with other drunks and by default, you'll surround yourself with all the drama and bullshit that goes with it.

A key factor in relapse is forgetting that while you are sober, there is an absence of problems. It's simple to see or feel something that is PRESENT: pain, drama, chaos, debt, guilt, regret, etc., but almost impossible to see the ABSENCE of those things. For instance, we can remember that we argued or behaved inappropriately when we were drinking, but we can't remember that we *don't do* those things while sober.

Relapse is often influenced by innocent sources; friends or family. Some people have no concept how destructive drinking might be for you. They may innocently say, "Oh you can have just one, what's the big deal?" There's no need for you to go into deep detail, but you have to emphatically say, "Thanks, but NO, I can't." People don't even have to offer you a drink for you to be influenced. Seeing friends and family drink socially can do it. My good friend Mike is an example. I admire his ability to drink one beer or 10 beers or no beers. He's able to stop or not drink whenever he wants. I see that and I wish I could do that but I realize that I can never be like that. I believe that is where many others relapse – they see the responsible drinker and think, "I could be like that." NO we can't, we're different. Doesn't mean we can't hang out with them or admire them.

The media is another example of innocent (covert) influence. The Dos Equis beer commercials about "The most interesting man in the world" are creative, entertaining & funny – but it's not reality. We cannot simultaneously be a rock star, baseball player, wealthy jetsetter, doctor, and drink beer all at the same time. However I will defend the media – breweries, distilleries and wineries are trying to sell a legal product – it is up to the individual to either buy or not buy the product. It is up to the individual to live responsibly.

"I can't help myself, I'm an alcoholic." That's weak and lame. That's blaming alcohol and alcohol can't defend itself. You have no control once alcohol is introduced into your bloodstream, but you do have control to make the conscious choice not to pour that first drop into your mouth.

Pay yourself a penalty: If you do happen to relapse, then pay yourself a penalty. This penalty should be large enough to make you never want to do it again – consider $100 as a minimum. You might be lucky enough where someone else doesn't make you pay a penalty; like the police and the court system or your spouse when they leave you. As I mentioned above, relapse does happen, but if there are no negative consequences, then it will keep happening and it will get easier to talk yourself into relapse. If you don't impose a hefty penalty upon yourself, eventually someone else will.

I had more fun as a drunk: I *thought* I was a lot of fun when I was drinking, but I didn't have to deal with me – I was me. When I first stopped drinking I felt as if all the fun had left from my life. At this writing I've been sober for more than 6 years. During these 6 years I've been re-learning what fun is for a sober person. Here's what I've noticed: There is a big variation between sober fun and drunk fun. Sober fun is different. I don't want to sound discouraging, but sober fun isn't as exciting as drunk fun, at least for me it's not. I've tried doing a lot of the same activities I used to do when I was drinking, they're just not as exciting. On the other hand, some activities *are* much more enjoyable and meaningful. They just don't seem the same.

It's kinda like explaining the difference between pleasure and happiness. Pleasure lasts only a fixed amount of time. Pleasure is a fleeting, physical feeling where happiness and joy is an emotion that lasts longer. It may not be as temporarily "orgasmic," but it becomes a way of being or feeling. So I can say that I am happier in life living sober, but I don't always seem to be having as much exciting fun.

When you're drunk, you laugh at the dumbest shit because it seems funny and sometimes you do the dumbest shit because it seems funny. But a lot of times when you're drunk, you can be laughing and having a blast and suddenly somebody says something or does something, then the next thing you know you're in a fight. Not necessarily a bar fight, but an argument with a friend or your spouse. That isn't fun is it?

So lemme talk about the fun of being sober. I have to consciously remind myself that I actually do have a lot of fun. It has required thought, time and numerous attempts at trying new things to find out what is fun, and even finding out what I don't like can be fun. The fun lies in the experience of discovery. When you sober up, you will have to re-learn how to have fun, and it can be learned. But it's harder to have sober fun than it is to have drunk fun. The primary reason is that once a mind altering substance like alcohol is introduced into your bloodstream it physically changes the way your brain interprets the stimuli that you're experiencing. For example, you can go to a comedy show or watch a comedy movie while you're drunk and laugh your ass off. But watch the same movie at home, sober, alone – you might not laugh that much or you might not think it's that funny. Drunken fun is far different than sober fun.

141

There are things that are still fun to do when sober and there are things that are actually more *enjoyable*. I'll give you my list of things that are fun and far more enjoyable sober, and hopefully it'll give you some ideas of fun things to do – or at least see them in a fun, new and enjoyable way. Number 1on the list is *sex*. There ain't nothing as good as sober sex. Some might say that it's fun to get all drunk, wild and crazy. But imagine getting all wild and crazy, and you can pay attention to what you're doing and you can vividly remember what you did. You'll be able to pay attention to your partner and you can learn about your partner and what your partner likes and you can understand your own body better. Try sober sex sometime… you may never have another drink again.

Another fun thing is going out to dinner sober. You can fully experience the meal and you won't have a bar bill that's more than the meal itself. Or make dinner with your spouse or date. You get time to talk and who knows what that can lead to? Going to the movies sober is fun – I can remember them and I can follow them better. I can pay attention and get involved in the plot development. Then there's traveling – seeing all the beauty of our country or the world through sober eyes is incredible. I'm amazed at all the stuff I missed when I travelled drunk. And there're so many other things which are still fun, enjoyable and much more meaningful. Working out, reading, golfing, gardening, going to strip joints, writing or talking with friends. I mentioned strip joints because I wanted to see if you were paying attention.

Try doing the things that you used to do, but when you do them now, pay attention to them. Don't just participate and do them, but experience them. Life is a 3-D movie that's playing right in front of you. Experience it. Don't get discouraged by sobriety if some stuff in life seems like it isn't fun anymore. Remember that sobriety is going to be completely different from what you're used to and different from what you might have expected out of it. If you figured that sobriety was going to be more fun and exciting than getting drunk, you're sadly mistaken. But it can be more enjoyable and meaningful than getting hammered. And as the old saying goes; would you rather get hammered or get nailed? Either way something's getting pounded. I would go for the latter.

Don't be a prisoner: I was once a slave to alcohol and now I'm a prisoner to it. I am not powerless over alcohol – because I don't drink it and it can't control me, but it still exerts a certain amount of power over me by controlling what I do, where I go and whom I hang out with. And that's the fucked up part – I'm strong enough to not introduce it into my bloodstream but it still plays a role in almost everything I do and how I think.

Alcohol is an inanimate object. It has no soul, mind or conscience, but it still has an influence over me. It's not doing this to me on purpose, *it* isn't trying to tease me, torture me or control me, I do this to myself. If I were to break it down logically, alcohol no longer has any physiological intoxicating power over me or what I do, but it does have that power over other people and some of those other people happen to be people that I would like to hang out with. So logically speaking, this should be easy to figure out – I don't drink it, so it can't influence my behavior, but it still does – it influences my emotions, my decisions and my life. I often feel powerless to the influences of alcohol around me. I've had to change what I do for entertainment and relaxation, and I've had to limit time spent with certain friends and I've even had to end some friendships – I mean holy shit – my marriage ended. So I am like a prisoner to alcohol, even though I don't drink it.

Even though you and I no longer drink, we can still be powerless and prisoners to alcohol by not doing the things we want, not going to the places we want to go to, or not spending time with the people we want to. A friend of mine attended AA for almost 10 years, he's now more than 12 years sober, but his sponsor would always tell him that he had to stay away from anywhere that served booze: bars, parties, restaurants, dance clubs, comedy clubs even bowling alleys. He wasn't supposed to do any of the things that might trigger a relapse. This guy loves to fish, and drinking was always part of fishing. That guy finally got sick and tired of living in a self-imposed prison. He said "fuck it" and started going out and doing things he enjoyed. That guy is **Jeff Nichols**, he's a SOBER comedian in New York, he's the author of the book "*Train Wreck*" and his book was made into a movie. Jeff will not allow alcohol to have power over his life and hold him back from doing the things he enjoys.

I'm not struggling with the concern that I'll crack or relapse if I hang around drinkers, I'm struggling with the reality that I'm limiting my own entertainment activities and I'm limiting some of my friendships because those other people drink. This isn't being imposed upon me and I'm not following the advice of a sponsor or doing what a group tells me to do. I'm doing this of my own volition and I can't blame anyone but myself.

I don't want to be a prisoner in my own insulated world. I need to find the right balance or at least practice more tolerance. Not tolerance for me to drink, but tolerance to accept that other people drink. To start drinking again so that I would "fit in" with the crowd would be foolish. To even attempt to be a social drinker would be my death sentence on the installment plan. I would fuck up every bit of progress I've made. This is one of the hard parts about living sober; to be controlled by and be a prisoner in a world of alcohol, even when you don't even drink it any more. Learn from me, don't be a prisoner to alcohol – be tolerant that others can and will drink and don't rob yourself of great friendships and fun things to do in life.

Summary: This chapter is a reminder for us hardcore drunks, that if you're thinking about trying to drink in moderation, it probably ain't gonna work for you. I wish it was different. I wish we could all enjoy a couple of drinks now and then, and then forget about it. But for some of us there is no middle ground. We either go balls-out and live to excess, or we must choose abstinence. If you never were a social drinker, you can't go back to something that you never were. However, if you can make moderation work for you, I truly do wish you the best of success with it.

Can I ever go back Worksheet:

Am I a prisoner to alcohol?: _____

Are there places I don't go, people I don't see because alcohol is there?:

_____

_____

Am I better off not going to those places or seeing those people? Why?:

_____

_____

_____

How will I protect my sobriety when I do venture out?: _____

_____

_____

If I ever relapse, what penalty would I pay myself?: _____

_____

_____

Has moderation ever worked for me in the past?: _____

Would moderation be any fun for me?: _____

If I were to moderate, how much would I limit myself to?: _____

_____

_____

_____

How would I enforce my moderation limits?: _____

_____

_____

_____

Have I ever seen moderation work for other drunks?: _____

Do I know anyone who tried moderation and failed?: _____

_____

What happened to them?: _____

_____

_____

Do I know people who moderate? Who are they?: _____

_____

_____

Arc they drunks or social drinkers? How do they do it?: _____

_____

_____

What can I learn from all this?: _____

_____

_____

#12) Not spreading the good word

"Who died and left you in charge?" – Anonymous

Not spreading the good word runs parallel to keeping your mouth shut and just acting normal. You will have your chance to help others, but you must first help yourself. After you've gotten yourself on track, the next people in line to help will be those who are closest to you. Not helping them see the light of sobriety, but helping them enjoy your sober life with you.

Spreading the good word of sobriety, trying to influence others into quitting drinking, or constantly talking about your new religion of sobriety (when you're not asked about it), will not improve your sober life nor make you a better person. There are appropriate times to talk about sober life skills. When those appropriate times occur (could be at an AA meeting, talking with someone who is seeking your help or is curious about how you do it), that's when the discussions will be of benefit to you. Going on a personal mission to convert the world to your new way of life won't endear you to your friends and family. Consider how excited you get when a Jehovah's Witness rings your doorbell (unless you're a Jehovah's Witness yourself – then you two goofs can stand there and talk all afternoon).

This book is about sober life skills, so this is the appropriate place to discuss it. If you met me out in public, regardless of whether it was a party, gym, grocery store, bar, picnic, wherever, I would not start talking with you about sobriety. Your life and what you do is none of my business. If it's a party or some other social event, I wouldn't even tell you that I write books about sobriety. If you asked me what I do for an occupation I would tell you, "I work in the field of behavioral studies – I study why I behave like an asshole." We'd both have a laugh and then I would ask about your life.

I'm not hiding what I do and I'm certainly not embarrassed. There is an appropriate time and setting to discuss sobriety work. From my own experience, people change as soon as I tell them what I do – especially if they're drinkers or are currently drinking in front of me. When I say "change" I mean that they reflexively think that I want to talk about sobriety and they unconsciously start discussing or defending their own drinking behavior. I don't give a fuck – I'm not there to judge. I want people to feel comfortable as themselves when they're around me, I want them to know that they can freely talk about whatever they want and behave however they want. So I'm better off when I don't disclose my sobriety and line of work, it allows the conversation and interaction to flow more naturally.

At some point you will be asked why you're not drinking (I'll give some sample responses to that question shortly), or the person may come right out and say, "Are you a recovering alcoholic?" Whether you like it or not, people do gossip, so someone may have *heard* that you're a recovered alcoholic. You have to gauge the setting and determine if it's appropriate to discuss it or not. No matter the setting, whenever I am asked, "Are you a recovering alcoholic?" I answer with, "No, I'm a Re-Invented Alcoholic." Typically a person will follow with, "What's a Re-Invented Alcoholic?" This changes the direction of the conversation. I now control the conversation and I don't have to defend my past behaviors – I can talk about my current plans and behaviors.

Do you need a title: People use titles as a quick way to establish who they are or what they do, i.e.; "I'm a teacher, I'm a Lutheran, I'm a Democrat." This gives them an identity. Some people also like to use the identifier of, "I'm a recovered alcoholic" as a way to gain attention or to subtly express some superiority. Even calling yourself a Re-Invented Alcoholic is an identifier. But do you really even need a title when it comes to talking about alcohol misuse and overuse?

Notice that I didn't call it alcoholism? Who gives a shit what you call it? You don't need to be clinically diagnosed an *alcoholic* to figure out if your drinking has created problems in your life, you already know. There is a wide variety of criteria and questions that need to be met for someone to be deemed a clinical alcoholic and different programs, disciplines and doctors use different criteria. You fill out one questionnaire and you're an alcoholic, fill out a different one and change an answer or two and you're not an alcoholic. But who cares if you get the "official diagnosis" as an alcoholic. Is that going to change anything? Is that going to change what's happened in your past or what's happening now? Probably not.

Receiving the title of *alcoholic* won't make any difference. When you do quit, do you then get a new title, like; recovering or recovered alcoholic? And when does someone go from recovering to recovered? "Well next Thursday I'll be recovered, but right now I'm still recovering." Or what if you quit, recover, relapse, recover again, and then go back to drinking? Are you an alcoholic squared? Holding a specific title isn't required. I'm sure that I will always crave alcohol and if I ever started drinking again, it would become a problem for me. So I guess you could say that I'm an alcoholic, even though I don't drink. So the title really means nothing. The only thing that counts are my actions. And the only thing that counts for you, are your actions. If you need to call yourself something, why not give yourself the title: **Re-Invented Alcoholic**.

151

Do yourself a favor, act normal: What is normal? Normal is acting and talking like a person who simply doesn't drink, but still engages in regular activities and conversation. I'm referring to just being yourself and talking about daily life with people. This can include entertainment gossip, political events, sports events, philosophy, religion, careers, families, relationships, hobbies, whatever. It's very tempting to want to always talk about sobriety, especially if you're newly sober. You can't help it because that's what you're mind is filled with. However, when you talk about everyday subjects, your mind is distracted from thinking about your sobriety. This helps you be more normal, it also allows other people to enjoy your company and be themselves around you, which will help you feel normal.

It's worth the effort to practice your conversation skills. A big part of conversation is listening to the other person. Let them talk, ask them questions, then listen to what they are saying. Pay attention to the subject at hand. It's easy to be listening to someone, they say something that reminds you of your drinking past, and you respond, "That's just like the time I was drunk and I screwed this up," or "That reminds me of a meeting I was at where this guys said..." Slow down your desire to interrupt or interject. Average conversations jump all over the map, from topic to topic. However, if whenever you add something to the conversation it always has something to do with your sobriety, people will quickly get tired of talking with you. So pay close attention to your own responses and your tone of voice.

I'm not saying that you ignore your thoughts or deny that you have them, but there are proper times and places to discuss alcohol issues. If the other person brings the subject up or expresses curiosity, then by all means talk about it. If it's someone you know and they know you fairly well, then you can discuss freely. If it's someone you just met, don't go into all the ugly details about the wreckage from your drinking.

Answers to inquiries: There will be times, when you expect it and least expect it, when someone offers you a drink. You don't have to get defensive and start preaching sobriety. Just say, "Thanks but I'm good" or lift up your glass of juice or bottle of water and say, "Thanks, I've already got one." What do you do if you're at a picnic and somebody walks right up to you and hands you an open, frosty bottle of beer? "Wow, that's really nice of you, but I'm good." Don't worry, it won't get wasted, somebody will drink it.

There will also be the curious questions that come in the form of: "How come you're not drinking? Don't you drink? Are you in recovery?" or some variation like that. People are just being inquisitive (or nosy). Many of us former drunks are tempted to spill our guts and talk about our recovery. If it's not the appropriate place or it's someone you just met, you're inviting some awkward conversation if you open up and start talking about sobriety. It has happened to me numerous times when I've answered honestly and told someone that I'm a former drunk. They start telling me how they hardly ever drink, or that they never drink during the week, blah, blah, blah (while they're holding a drink in their hand). This is why I now give evasive answers. You are not obligated to answer honestly. So what if you lie – this is your life and your sobriety. You can simply answer with, "I don't feel like it," or "I don't drink anymore, I really don't feel like talking about it." Avoid the temptation to spill your guts or spread the good word.

The Big Business of alcohol: I believe that an important element of enjoying your sobriety is gaining an understanding of the alcohol industries. When you understand and respect these businesses, you won't hate alcohol, which will help you not spread the good word. In fact, instead of talking about sobriety or recovery, you will be in a position to intelligently discuss the many aspects of alcohol and its effects on the economy.

So let's look at the big business of alcohol. On one side of the street there's a drug and alcohol rehabilitation facility and right across the street is a bar. It might seem like they're competing with one another for customers, in some ways they are, but without each other neither business would exist. And this freedom is what fuels the big business of alcoholism. Billions of dollars are spent by people on getting drunk and billions are spent by people going to rehab trying to get and stay sober. I believe that's how it should be – we should have these choices in a free economy. I have the freedom to turn left into the parking lot of the bar or to turn right into the parking lot of the rehab center. Neither of these businesses is morally better than the other. Bars and alcohol exist for people's entertainment; bars and liquor stores charge for it. Rehabilitation facilities are there to help people with their alcohol problem and most of them charge for it. Those who sell alcohol are supplying people with a product that they want. Then there's the rehabilitation business and they are also supplying people with a service that they want.

The alcohol industry has a major influence on our economy both good and bad. The financial devastation that would occur if everyone suddenly stopped drinking is incalculable. Your own job probably in some strange circuitous way has something to do with the alcohol industry. Without that industry there would be mass unemployment. Let me use beer as an example.

We start with the farmers who grow the wheat, barley and hops. Those farmers buy tractors, fuel, fertilizer, storage bins, etc. Once harvested those raw materials need to be transported to the brewery using rail systems and trucking. At the brewery you have thousands of employees making the beer, using machinery and equipment that someone else manufactured. The finished product is then put into bottles, cans, kegs, etc. All of those products were made by someone else. Then there's the packaging, which was made by someone else. The final product is then distributed to bars, restaurants, liquor stores and grocery stores. The sale of the final product employs bartenders, store workers, waitresses, etc. Let's not forget about how much of that beer is sold at concerts, fairs, festivals and professional sports venues.

This is not an argument in support of YOU drinking; it's just an honest and realistic appreciation of the beer industry. If every Re-Invented Alcoholic tried to talk everyone into quitting drinking (and we were successful), many of us would end up unemployed.

Alcohol also has negative implications on our economy. It's impossible to determine how much revenue is lost due to employees calling in "sick" or performing poorly at work due to a hangover. There is no way to measure the costs to health insurers for accidents, illnesses and injuries resulting from drunkenness. Law enforcement generates a lot of revenue from drunk drivers, but it also requires more manpower to combat drunk drivers. Then there is the cost to families and individuals whose drinking brings wreckage that cannot be counted in monetary value.

Wow, I've been all over the map here. Lemme wrap up the big business of alcohol and alcoholism. The goal of the beer, wine and liquor companies is to sell you their product. That's fine, that's called capitalism. Used within moderation these products can be fun. When it's overused and it becomes a problem, that's where the big business of rehab comes into play. I find it fascinating that we juicers spend billions of dollars trying to get drunk, then we spend billions of dollars on law enforcement to stop us from driving drunk, and then spend billions more battling medical ailments due to being drunk and then spend a few more billion on trying to stay sober. And that is precisely why I love America so much – because I have the freedom of choice – I can choose to drink or not drink, I can choose my own self-destruction or I can choose to fulfill my life. And only I can make those choices for myself.

What's the point of my little discussion here? I believe that when you understand the importance of alcohol in our economy and the role it plays in society, you will be less likely to hate alcohol and will become more tolerant of others who do drink. You won't make it your personal mission to lecture everyone about the evils of alcohol. I believe this will aid you in being normal and enjoying all that life has to offer - you just happen to be a non-drinker.

You might think I'm cheating because I've used some excerpts from my other book. Hey the shit is relevant. Why try and rewrite what is applicable here? I happen to think the raw way I present things is beneficial in certain situations. This segment is excerpted from Chapter #12 of *Living Sober Sucks*.

> Just to let you know, a lot of people will act and treat you differently when they find out that you *used* to be a drinker. They will make references about drinking or joke about drinking, then become self-conscious when they remember that you're a *"recovering alcoholic"* and then apologize for their insensitivity. I noticed that when I have told people who are drinking that I don't drink any more they get uncomfortable and say things like, "I could quit anytime I want to," or, "I'm not an alcoholic, I never drink before work." Well guess what - I don't give a fuck - I don't want to talk about that.

> In social settings where alcohol is being served, don't be the one who opens the door by announcing, "I am a recovering alcoholic." You would be treated more normally if you said, "I'm a recovering rapist, but I'm getting better." (At least they wouldn't talk with you about it.) And don't comment about other's drinking. Who are you to judge? Keep in mind that no amount of lecturing on the evils of alcohol or criticizing how much someone else

drinks will help make you a better person or keep you from drinking. Just because you think that getting sober helped your life doesn't mean it will be good for anybody else. An important element of your new sober life is that you *don't preach the good news* unless you are asked about it. I know it's exciting to have found a *new religion*, but don't bore people with it. You might as well walk into a stag party and say, "Hi everybody, who wants to talk about Jesus?" People will more than likely end up knowing that you're an ex-drinker anyway. Whether you like it or not, people like to talk and gossip. Don't be surprised or offended if someone asks you how your recovery is going. Some people may avoid you because they aren't sure what to say to you. Some might stare - because they think former alcoholics are freaks. Who cares what other people think - you can't control their thoughts - you can only control your own. I am guilty myself of being uncertain of how to approach a newly recovered drunk. A good friend of mine informed me that his wife had gone through alcohol treatment. When I saw her at a graduation party I didn't know what to say at first. Should I ask her about it? Should I offer my input? I opted to quit worrying about her and pay attention to my own thoughts and actions.

It is easy to find yourself going to the anti-alcohol extreme. You certainly don't want people avoiding you or not inviting you to social events, parties, bar mitzvahs or poetry readings. (Well I guess it would be okay if they didn't invite me to poetry readings.) Parties, bars, weddings and picnics are no place to discuss your newfound lifestyle. If someone asks you how you sobered up or wants to talk about it, tell them to buy my book.

Okay, seriously, talk casually with them or say something like, "I don't know if this is the best time or place to talk about this. We can get together for lunch or I can call you later and we can talk a bit more freely then." Use your judgment. Be smart. If it's an A.A. function, a religious function or a specified non-alcohol function, then the subject is probably welcome.

This is excerpted from Chapter #11 of *Living Sober Sucks*.

Step #12 - "Having had a spiritual awakening as a result of these steps, we tried to carry this message to alcoholics, and to practice these principles in all our affairs." This whole step rubs me wrong. I had no "spiritual awakening" (I don't think God likes me anyway). I came to my own conclusions on the benefits of sobriety. I honestly accept the good and bad consequences of my actions. You can call it an "awakening" but this came only after I was physically cleared of alcohol.

I understand that this principle states that we should carry the message to other alcoholics. What message? That they should become a member of a recovery group or embrace my sober way of life? I will not force my philosophy or my way of life upon anyone. If someone wants to talk with me about alcoholism I will do so, if someone wants my help, I will always offer it, otherwise I mind my own business. The best way that I can carry the message is to live sober. True, I wrote this book and I run LivingSoberSucks.com but these are intended for those who are actively seeking help. I don't go around lecturing people on the ills of alcoholism. I want to be a welcome guest wherever I go. I let people do what they want and let them get as drunk as they want. If their drinking bothers me, then I don't hang out with them. I worry about myself and just live sober.

Summary: If you want to live a *normal* life, do not make spreading the good word of sobriety your personal mission. You will only alienate yourself from others who are not interested in your message and you will only insulate yourself with others who already agree with your message. You will have your chance to share with others. When you live by example, other people (but not everyone) will begin to ask you about sobriety. If you are compelled to discuss and engage in conversations about sobriety, do it at the proper times and appropriate places. Go to AA meetings; get involved in community or religious support programs.

Remember that everyone has the freedom and right to believe whatever they want, regardless of whether you agree with them or not. If you live in the United States, you and I have freedom of choice. If you're over 21, you have the legal right to enjoy the legal product called alcohol. You and I also have the freedom to destroy our own lives with that product.

It is solely up to you to decide if and how you want to live as a sober person. Study, research, ask questions, gct involved and be a participant in your sobriety. Make the best out of this. No one else will or can do it for you. You can lean on others, you can turn to others for help, but you will have to do this yourself.

Not spreading the word Worksheet:

What do I tell people when they ask why I no longer drink?: _____

_____

_____

Do I have a title?: _____

Do I need a title?: _____

Do I flaunt my non-drinker status?: _____

Do I talk more about my drinking history and wreckage than necessary?:

_____

Do I push my thoughts about sobriety onto other people?: _____

Do I think poorly of other people who drink, am I judgmental of them?:

_____

How can I be of help to others who ask about living sober?: _____

_____

_____

How can I be of more help to MYSELF with my own sobriety?: _____

_____

_____

_____

Closing thoughts

"When all else fails I turn to me – I am who I'm stuck with."
Mark A. Tuschel

his book is not the final answer to all your questions. Living sober is a constant evolutionary process. Every situation is different, every former drunk is different. My intention is to get you to think and help you help yourself. There is no rhyme or relevant sequence to these closing thoughts. They are random statements which I believe are appropriate in closing this book.

● I don't expect everyone to like me or agree with me. If I try to be everything to everyone, I will be nothing to no one – including myself.

● If reading this book incites people to discuss, disagree and engage in debate about alcohol control, then I have accomplished my goal. That goal is to get others to think.

● Living sober and enjoying sobriety isn't always that easy but it can be rewarding. Please don't ever give up on yourself.

● It's not always a question of, "What am I doing wrong?" It's more constructive to ask, "What can I do more of that's right?"

● A favorite saying is, "It's never too late to start." That's true, but I prefer to say, "It's never too early to start." Don't wait for everything to align just right before you begin your Re-Invention. You've already started just by no longer drinking and by reading this book. It will now be up to you whether you take action or not.

● I learn from talking to and watching other people. I learn what I want to be like and what I don't want to be like.

● Gonna start living sober? Don't expect ANYTHING out of sobriety – expect EVERYTHING from yourself.

● Problems aren't the cause of drinking; drinking is the cause of problems.

● When I wake up, I have to go to my job as a sober person. The more I work at my job, the better I get at it. But like any job, sometimes I'd rather be doing something else. Some days my job sucks. So??? And just like having a job, sobriety is my own personal responsibility – to show up on time, get better at what I do, further my education about my job and to do good work. I choose what job I apply for; therefore I also choose my sobriety. Nobody forces me to work, to drink or to live sober.

● In the end, most of us, if not all of us, are incentivized by *personal benefits* - to gain something or to avoid losing something. Even altruistic acts are for our own benefit. Behavioral change typically doesn't occur until a significant price must be paid for our actions. Sadly, sometimes it's too late to pay any price.

- Fear elicits REACTION while reward promotes ACTION. When someone sobers up out of fear or has fear/coercion thrust upon them, i.e.: "You're powerless, you're flawed, you're a bad person because you're an alcoholic, you're arrested," that is when their behavior will be reactive. They do things based on what they think they should do at that moment. When someone sobers up out of desire for reward, they are propelled to undertake action; moral, ethical and positive action to maintain survival. Reaction is a short-lived activity simply to get someone off your back. Reward (for yourself and for those you care about) causes you to have a long-term view of sobriety.

- Success is not just lots of money (it doesn't hurt to have lots of money). Success is: Being respected, being a good parent, being faithful to your spouse/partner, being true to yourself, being proud of yourself, doing the small things. Not cheating, lying or stealing when you have the opportunity. Success is easier than you think.

Acknowledgements

"If I spend all my time with myself, the only opinions I would ever hear would be my own." – Mark A. Tuschel

There are so many people in my life that must be acknowledged for their help. There are those who have spent their time and talents reviewing and editing this work. Not only are they skilled editors*, they are friends. I would like to give them public recognition: Jhennifer Menting, Linda Bryl, Dana Meredith, Jeff Kolby. There are also numerous other friends who spent their time discussing this project and the various subjects. Every one of you has helped open my eyes up to so many additional areas of making the best out of sobriety.

I acknowledge the friends who stand by me and care about me. The ones who say to me "Quit working for a few minutes and enjoy what you have earned." When they say "earned," they're not just referring to money, but to the joys of friendship and relaxation. They engaged me in spirited conversations, debating with me about religion, politics, financial markets, capitalism, education, human behavior, dating, you name it. You challenge my mind.

I also want to acknowledge all the people who don't like me and don't care about me. Not the random public, but anyone who ever said that I couldn't stay sober and would never amount to anything. "Thanks." You keep me going. I must also acknowledge those in the general public who don't agree with me. They help keep me in check. They help me question my premises. Not question my beliefs and principles, but to check my data. By questioning my premises I am required to study more and ultimately gain more knowledge.

167

The most important people to acknowledge are those who call or email me and say, "I have been searching for something like this. I am so grateful for you sharing your stories. I feel wonderful about what **I am doing for myself and my family**. I am actually proud of myself." That's gratifying to me. To know that something I put out into the world inspired another person to take control of their own life and be proud about it.

Finally, as arrogant as this may sound, I wish to acknowledge myself. Without self-discipline, effort and conscious planning, I would still be drunk (or dead) today. I am proud of myself.

No one else can make you proud; you have to do it yourself. Go do something that you can be proud of.

I sincerely wish that your life turns out better than you ever imagined,

Mark A. Tuschel

*(Note regarding editors: Any spelling, grammar or punctuation mistakes in this book are not a reflection on the editors. They are smarter than I am. I had the final say in the wording, layout and punctuation of this book. Any errors that you the reader notice are completely my own responsibility.)

Mark Tuschel is also the author of:

Living Sober Sucks *(but living drunk sucks more)*

The Malingerer's Handbook – Living off the fruits of someone else's labor

Contact information:

Mark@livingsobersucks.com

www.LivingSoberSucks.com